SAUNDERS

2017

2016

DATE DUE

s in

ool

ent

ner

Wit

MSN, RN, CNS, PHN

ELSEVIER

ELSEVIER

3251 Riverport Lane
St. Louis, Missouri 63043

SAUNDERS GUIDE TO SUCCESS IN NURSING SCHOOL, 2016-2017
A STUDENT PLANNER, 12TH EDITION   ISBN: 978-0-323-44372-2

Notices

Knowledge and best practice in this field are constantly changing. As new research and experience broaden our understanding, changes in research methods, professional practices, or medical treatment may become necessary.

Practitioners and researchers must always rely on their own experience and knowledge in evaluating and using any information, methods, compounds, or experiments described herein. In using such information or methods they should be mindful of their own safety and the safety of others, including parties for whom they have a professional responsibility.

With respect to any drug or pharmaceutical products identified, readers are advised to check the most current information provided (i) on procedures featured or (ii) by the manufacturer of each product to be administered, to verify the recommended dose or formula, the method and duration of administration, and contraindications. It is the responsibility of practitioners, relying on their own experience and knowledge of their patients, to make diagnoses, to determine dosages and the best treatment for each individual patient, and to take all appropriate safety precautions.

To the fullest extent of the law, neither the Publisher nor the authors, contributors, or editors, assume any liability for any injury and/or damage to persons or property as a matter of products liability, negligence or otherwise, or from any use or operation of any methods, products, instructions, or ideas contained in the material herein.

Library of Congress Cataloging-in-Publication Data

Names: DeWit, Susan C., author.
Title: Saunders guide to success in nursing school 2016-2017 : a student planner / Susan C. deWit.
Other titles: Saunders student nurse planner 2014-2015 | Guide to success in nursing school 2016-2017
Description: 12th edition. | St. Louis, Missouri : Elsevier, [2017] | Preceded by Saunders student nurse planner 2015-2016 / Susan C. deWit. 11th edition. 2016. | Includes bibliographical references and index.
Identifiers: LCCN 2015051239 | ISBN 9780323443722 (pbk.)
Subjects: | MESH: Nursing Process | Patient Care Planning | Medical Records | Students, Nursing
Classification: LCC RT73 | NLM WY 100 | DDC 610.73076–dc23 LC record available at http://lccn.loc.gov/2015051239

Senior Vice President and Director: Loren Wilson
Senior Content Strategist: Nancy O'Brien
Content Development Manager: Ellen Wurm-Cutter
Associate Content Development Specialist: Erin Garner
Publishing Services Manager: Hemamalini Rajendrababu
Project Manager: Janish Ashwin Paul
Design Direction: Patrick Ferguson

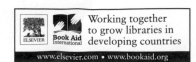

Working together
to grow libraries in
developing countries

ELSEVIER   Book Aid International

Printed in United States of America

Last digit is the print number: 9 8 7 6 5 4 3 2 1

www.elsevier.com • www.bookaid.org

To the memory of

Julia Catherine Reaves,

my mentor, friend, and former teaching partner,
who provided the foundation for many of the ideas
that appear in this book to help students.
Catherine's dedication to nursing, to students, and to holistic
health care for the elderly provided continuing inspiration.

To all my colleagues who have helped me decide throughout the
editions of this book what would be most useful to nursing students:
Barbara Michaels, EdD, MSN, Kathy Pritchett, MSN,
Kay O'Neal, MSN, Holly Stromberg, MSN,
and Jimmie Borum, MSN.

PREFACE

The student nursing experience is one of the most complex in the undergraduate curriculum. It entails not only the class work and home study common to all undergraduate programs but also unique clinical preparations and experiences. In talking with students, nursing program administrators, and nursing classroom and clinical instructors, we found that people were looking for a guide to help students plan and organize their time and information, particularly with respect to the clinical experience. Much of the material in this book is for quick reference throughout the nursing program and during clinical experiences.

CLINICAL INFORMATION

Chapters 1 through 6 of this planner include an orientation to and a guide for success throughout your nursing program, including suggestions for getting the most from clinical rotations, achieving success in distance learning courses, dealing with stress, and a broad array of useful data and procedures. The information in this section was selected especially for student use in a quick reference format and has been indexed for user convenience.

CALENDARS

Yearly, monthly, and weekly calendars have been included so that students can plan their short-term weekly activities and long-term projects and goals.

CONTENTS

5 Clinical Quick Reference, 82

SUCCESS IN NURSING SCHOOL

■ QUALIFICATIONS AND PREPARATION

Nursing schools generally have some prerequisites that must be passed before entry into the nursing program. Check with your school regarding the requirements and scheduling of the required courses.

Specific regulations and requirements exist for any person who has had a criminal conviction or been treated for a psychiatric occurrence. **It is wise to check with your state board of nursing before beginning the nursing program or during the first course to review these regulations and requirements.** Even juvenile offenses are not sealed to the Board of Nursing. Licensure may be denied because of past offenses that are "substantially related to health care" or exhibit a lack of integrity such as bouncing checks or shoplifting. If there is a past criminal history of offenses, character references may counter juvenile offenses.

Clinical agencies require a background check that includes drug screening as for all employees and volunteers before a student is allowed into the clinical area.

■ ETHICS AND PROFESSIONALISM

In its *Code of Ethics for Nurses with Interpretive Statements*, the American Nurses Association (ANA) states, "Ethics is an integral part of the foundation of nursing. Nursing has a distinguished history of concern for the welfare of the sick, injured, and vulnerable and for social justice" (ANA, 2001). Nursing students are expected to act ethically **at all times**. Acting ethically includes being honest with your written work and tests and following the policies of the institution in which you are a student. It means protecting the privacy and well-being of your patient at all times with adherence to the Health Insurance Portability and Accountability Act (HIPAA) privacy law. Acting ethically also relates to your **personal** life as well. It is important to act with integrity and pay attention to what you say and do.

Professionalism means that you act decorously, with good manners, and treat others courteously. An example is to change out of your uniform before going out with friends after clinical or work for drinks or boisterous activity. When blogging or commenting on social networking sites, remember that what you post is no longer in your control and can be seen by anyone. Privacy settings on social networking sites are easy to circumvent and are often changed by web administrators without notice. It is possible that the information you thought you were sharing with close friends has been viewed by teachers and prospective employers. It is not appropriate to use these venues for venting about school issues or other people. It is not professional to use coarse language orally or in writing on social networking sites. **Employers often check these sites to gather data about the character**

of prospective employees. A guide to basic good manners is available at http://www.nursingcenter.com/lnc/journalarticle?Article_ID=983314.

Cell phones must be turned off completely during class time. In the clinical areas, cell phones are to be used only to contact your instructor.

■ CHALLENGES OF NURSING SCHOOL

Nursing school is an exciting and challenging adventure that demands significant time and energy. Because nursing is a discipline comprising knowledge from many related fields, you are asked to learn to think critically, synthesize information, and then apply this information to everyday situations involving people. To learn to care correctly and safely for people who are ill, you must learn a large amount of information in a relatively short time. This process requires an efficient use of time and resources.

On Campus

SYLLABUS

A course outline or syllabus will be provided for each nursing course (Figure 1-1). This outline or syllabus may be available on the college intranet platform for you to download and print or available for purchase in the bookstore or handed out in class. Becoming familiar with the entire layout of each course is the first step after you acquire the syllabus. Syllabi, or course outlines, are usually divided into units of study that contain a list of learning objectives. A correlated outline of the content to be covered in the unit and related learning opportunities or activities may also be provided. The latter usually includes textbook and journal reading assignments, multimedia presentations, compact discs (CDs) or online instruction modules, clinical simulations, and suggestions for review of material covered in earlier prerequisite classes, such as anatomy and physiology.

The syllabus, or other class materials on the school intranet or handed out at the first class meeting, will state policies regarding attendance requirements, student behavior in class and clinical areas, grading criteria, dress code for clinical areas, grievance procedures, and other topics. A list of required texts and a statement about evaluation of performance for the course will be provided. Many schools are switching to electronic textbooks and therefore require students to have an iPad, tablet, or other electronic device to access texts.

SCHOOL PHILOSOPHY AND STUDENT RESPONSIBILITY

Each school and nursing program has a statement of philosophy that explains how the school and instructors view the student, teacher, and learning. Most schools expect the student to be an active learner and the teacher to be a facilitator of learning. This means that you must take responsibility for your own learning and must not depend on instructors to provide all the knowledge you need to pass a particular course. You are expected to participate in all classroom and lab activities.

Students who use English as a second language must be able to read and write in English by writing or printing in blue or black ink as well as by computer keyboard.

For this reason, going to class prepared for the topics to be covered that day is very important. You are properly prepared if you have read the text pages relative to the content to be covered, taken study notes, considered the objectives to be

Sample Page from a Nursing Course Syllabus

Content Outline	Learning Objectives	Assignment	Learning Resources

Unit 2 Assessment
A. Introduction
B. History taking
  1. History of current problems
  2. Medical history
  3. Psychosocial data
C. Physical Assessment
  1. Assessment Techniques
    a. Observation
    b. Palpation
    c. Percussion
    d. Auscultation
    e. Olfaction
  2. Height and weight
  3. Neurologic Assessment
    a. Level of consciousness
    b. Pupillary response
    c. Motor/sensory response
  4. Vital sign trends
    d. Testing visual acuity
  5. Assisting for a medical exam
    a. Positioning
    b. Draping
	1. Demonstrate methods for obtaining a health history from a patient.
	
	2. Describe the steps in performing a chart review.
	
	3. Identify techniques used for obtaining physical assessment data.
	
	4. List the equipment needed for a complete physical assessment.
	
	5. Correctly demonstrate a basic neurologic assessment.
	
	6. Identify indications of a patient problem from vital sign trends.
	
	7. Prepare a patient for a medical physical examination, including a rectal and pelvic examination.
		deWit Fundamentals Chapters 21 and 22.
		
		Potter & Perry Skills & Techniques Chapters 17 and 18
		
		Simulation practice in Skill Lab
			Evolve text Web site
			  Video clips
			  Mosby's Nursing Skills
			    Video Exercises
			
			Mosby's Nursing Skills Video/CD-ROM:
			  Measurements Video: Height and weight; intake and output; vital signs.
			
			Article: Murthy, TVSP. (2009) A new score to validate coma in emergency department—FOUR score. *Indian Journal of Neurotrauma, 6*(1), 59-61.

FIGURE 1-1 Sample page from a nursing course syllabus.

covered, viewed voice-over PowerPoint or recorded lectures on the intranet if available, and noted questions that should be asked in class.

During orientation to each course, the calendar of when course material will be covered by date will be given. Test dates and assignment due dates will also be set. Enter this information in the calendar section of this planner or into a tablet or smartphone calendar. Doing so assists in organizing time and study activity.

CAMPUS RESOURCES

Become acquainted with the resources on campus that can make life easier. All nursing students have access to the learning resource center or library. Your campus might also have a learning or tutoring center, adult resource center for single parents or students with special needs, office for students with disabilities, counseling center, computer lab, testing center, media room, skills and simulation lab, and student center. You should become familiar with the school intranet system, where syllabi, class notes, instructions, announcements for class, and other information may be posted. The intranet platform and software shell (e.g., Blackboard, WebCT, Intranet, E-College, etc.) that the school uses should have a tutorial available to help you navigate the site and areas within it you will need. The school catalog or student handbook describes these areas and services. Plan time to seek out, visit, and use the services and areas that could be useful to you. You are entitled to the services offered through the tuition and fees paid for courses. Your school may have a bulletin board that features important announcements and reminders for nursing students.

Schedule time each week for working with library references, using available media, participating in computer or mannequin simulations, and practicing skills. Few schools can schedule sufficient lab time for students to learn a skill thoroughly or provide adequate practice time to master a skill. **You are expected to practice on your own time.** Schedule these activities each week in the calendar section of this planner. Practice with a peer, and when the skill is mastered, ask your peer to evaluate your performance critically. Peer evaluation will help ensure that you are ready for instructor "check-off" evaluation.

SKILL LAB OR SIMULATION PRACTICE

You should prepare for lab time by studying the assigned skill before coming to the lab. If media presentations are available, use them. Be attentive to instruction in the lab, and practice the skill using a guide and a partner to check your technique. There may be a pretest and then a post-test for the exercises or scenarios.

A simulation experience with a mannequin may take the place of some clinical hours and is just as serious a learning experience as clinical experience with a real patient. The mannequins are programmed to react to a given situation or problem much like a person would react. You are expected to treat the simulation mannequin as you would a real human. To prepare for a simulation assignment, you should find out the following:

- Are there preparation assignments?
- What are the objectives for the experience?
- What is the dress code?
- What kind of orientation to the equipment will be given?
- What should you bring to the simulation area?
- Will the simulation exercise be recorded?
- Is confidentiality about the simulation exercise required?

At the Hospital

The term *clinical* refers to the time you are scheduled to learn at the hospital or another clinical site. When you have learned the preliminary skills necessary to function in the clinical area, you will be assigned to a clinical facility. Hospitals, long-term care facilities (nursing homes), mental health facilities, home health agencies, school health offices, and outpatient clinics are all referred to as *clinical facilities*. Clinical rotations may be for 1 or 2 days, a few weeks, half of a semester, or a full semester. Sometimes night or weekend shift times are assigned. Once assigned to a clinical facility, you may be given data about the type of patient assignment the day before the clinical experience is to take place. Otherwise, specific patients are assigned at the beginning of the clinical session.

Hospital rules usually require that tattoos and piercing jewelry not be visible on student nurses. Cell phone use on the units is restricted to contacting your instructor for assistance. Only the items you need for your clinical assignment are to be brought into the hospital. Purses and other personal items should be locked in the trunk of your vehicle. Lockers are not usually available for students. The hospital usually insists on photo ID and may take your picture for your badge that will give you access to the units to which your clinical group is assigned.

CLINICAL ORIENTATION

During clinical orientation you will be given an overview of the facility, including its size, general services, and the community it serves; whether the facility is a public or private business; its administrative structure; the physical layout; and the areas to which you will be assigned. A description of the type of nursing care used on the units will be provided. Some hospitals use a team nursing approach, some use managed care, and others use primary nursing; many different types of care delivery exist. (The types of care delivery are discussed further in your fundamentals of nursing course.) Importantly, you must understand the division of labor among the personnel on the unit, the organization of the unit, and the lines of communication. **Note that the patient, or client, is considered the customer and is to be treated as such.**

A clinical facility orientation checklist is provided to help you prepare to care for patients and to feel more comfortable in the environment of the assigned clinical unit (Box 1-1). This checklist is most appropriate for a hospital unit, but it can be adapted to other types of clinical facilities.

PATIENT ASSIGNMENT

During clinical orientation, your instructor will describe how you will receive your patient assignments for the clinical days; either your instructor will assign patients to you or you will choose your own patients. In either case, you will need to gather data to prepare for your patient assignment. Box 1-2 provides a checklist for you to use to be certain you gather the essential information.

HEAVILY TRAFFICKED AREAS

During orientation you should pay attention to heavily trafficked areas to avoid obstructing the work of the unit. Heavily traveled pathways and chairs where nurses or physicians need to sit to document should be avoided at peak times of the day. Consideration will be appreciated. If the facility has not completely changed to electronic medical records and is using paper charts, whenever a chart is taken away from the immediate area of the nurses' station, inform the unit

BOX 1-1

Clinical Facility Orientation

MEET THE PERSONNEL AND FACILITY DEPARTMENTS

Note phone numbers of essential people and departments:

- Unit director's or charge nurse's name (or both) and their telephone numbers
- Staff nurses', case managers', and nursing assistants' names
- Physicians' names for assigned patients
- Type of unit
- Dietary department
- Pharmacy
- Radiology (x-ray) department
- Physical therapy department
- Respiratory therapy department
- Rapid response for a code team
- Central supply room or central stores
- Surgery control desk
- Instructor (cell or pager)

EQUIPMENT

- Learn to work the intercom system if students are allowed to use it.
- Use colored light system or other types of designations for special patient needs.
- Learn to obtain forms with patient identification.
- Review the procedure for using the fire extinguishers and note alarm locations.
- Proceed to a patient unit and perform the following:
  - Operate all of the light switches.
  - Turn the television and radio on and off, and adjust the volume; use the other functions of the TV unit. Note patient education programs available on the facility intranet.
  - Raise and lower the whole bed; raise the head and then the foot.
  - Raise and lower the side rails.
  - Open and close the curtains.
  - Practice using the call-light system.
  - Adjust the shower or bath controls.
- Learn how to document activities on the computer; note your password for the computer for documentation of activities and notes.

ENVIRONMENT

- Explore the layout of the nurses' station, and find extra forms if the system is not paperless. Find items you may need during a clinical day:
  - Chart rack (if charts are used)
  - Kardex or computer patient care sheets
  - Drug reference access
  - Policy and procedure manuals
  - Dietary manual
  - Communication board
  - Out-of-the-way areas where students can sit to chart
  - Location of computers for documentation and access to the Internet and clinical agency system
- Find all supplies that you may need for patient care; explore the supply cart and various cupboards.
- Find the clean linen storage area.
- Locate the dirty linen disposal area and the utility room.
- Locate the lift equipment locations.

Clinical Facility Orientation (cont'd)

- Find where the scales are kept.
- Find the staff restroom.
- Locate the patient shower or tub bathrooms if such exist on the unit.
- Find the room where reports are given.
- Determine where to leave your coat.
- Inquire where the student–patient assignment sheets are posted.

PROCEDURES

- Learn how to access the EMR and other patient data in the computer, if permitted.
- Determine how to document care (check the documentation manual).
- Understand the fire or disaster procedures.
- Learn the procedure for initiating the emergency code for cardiac or respiratory arrest.
- Determine how to handle hazardous materials.
- Understand the procedures for ordering supplies for patient care and for posting charges for supplies and equipment used.
- Learn how to administer medication and to use the medication-dispensing machine.
- Understand the procedure for charting as-needed (*pro re nata* [PRN]) medications and one-time doses.
- Learn the narcotic checkout procedure and the use of the automated dispensing machine.
- Understand the special charting and reporting procedures (e.g., elevated vital signs, change in condition).

secretary where the chart will be in case someone needs it. Charts must be replaced exactly where they were found.

Establishing *paperless* hospitals is a priority, which means that within the next several years, facilities will use electronic rather than paper medical records. Students must become adept at accessing information about their patients via computer.

Take note of particular landmarks on the way to the assigned unit if the facility is large or the layout is confusing. Try to travel to and from the unit on the same elevators each time, and note hallway decor and signs with unit and room number designations.

Some instructors will assign you to a staff nurse the first day of clinical orientation to ensure that you can become more comfortable and learn the usual routine of the unit.

PRECONFERENCE AND POSTCONFERENCE

Many schools have a preconference period at the beginning of the clinical day to provide an opportunity for students to clarify assignments, ask questions, and gather moral support for the day. At the end of the clinical day, most schools have a 30-minute to several hour clinical postconference time for discussion of the day's events, sharing of experiences, and instructor-guided learning to help meet the week's objectives. Students are often asked to make presentations on short topics, complete quizzes, or participate in group learning activities. Sometimes speakers are invited to present special topics to the clinical group.

Clinical Assignment Information Form

BOX 1-2

- Diagnoses
- Surgery and date performed
- Current vital signs and condition; vital sign schedule
- Daily weight required?
- Diet:
  - Intake and output (I&O)
- Activity allowed:
  - Degree of mobility
  - Traction
- Type of bath required
- Tubes:
  - Intravenous (IV)
  - Nasogastric (NG)
  - Foley
  - Drains
  - Other
- Pain:
  - Control method
  - Pain score
- Medications
- Allergies
- Risk areas:
  - Skin
  - Falls
- Treatments:
  - Dressing changes
  - Thromboembolic deterrent (TED) hose
  - Heat or cold
  - Sitz baths
  - Incentive spirometer
  - Sequential compression devices (SCDs)
- Therapies:
  - Physical
  - Occupational
  - Respiratory
  - Turn, cough, and deep breathe (TCDB)
  - Speech
- Tests ordered
- Equipment in use
- Prostheses
- Losses:
  - Hearing
  - Vision (wears glasses or contact lenses)
  - Paralysis or limb weakness
- Communication:
  - Problems
  - Language spoken

NETWORKING

You should begin networking with classmates and other nursing students as soon as school starts. Networking will help you find out what to expect in other courses, at particular clinical facilities, and from particular instructors. Networking is also a way to develop study buddies and to set up a study group. Online groups of student nurses provide a social network for those with little time to socialize otherwise. Joining the student nurses' association (SNA) at your school is one way to begin. Your instructors can provide you with information about SNA meetings and contact information for sponsors and officers.

■ SETTING UP FOR SUCCESS

Being successful in nursing school requires good time management, efficient study skills, and proper use of appropriate resources. Nursing students often have to juggle family responsibilities, work, and school, along with the miscellaneous tasks of daily life. **The key to success is careful planning and as much simplification as possible in all areas of your life for the duration of the nursing program.** Beside the hours spent in class and in clinical settings, a rule of thumb for planning study time is 2 hours per week for each credit hour of the course to achieve a passing grade. In other words, for a 3-credit-hour course, you will need to spend 6 hours studying per week to obtain a C average.

Organizing Your Time

WEEKLY TIME MAP

Coordinating all of your responsibilities and activities of day-to-day life with your school class and study schedule is essential to your success in any nursing program. Making a weekly time map in which you map out the time required for everything from cooking dinner or mowing the yard to picking up the children from school is a good way to coordinate all responsibilities and activities. The student living alone will want to coordinate time for friends, exercise, and favorite pastimes with the school schedule. The student living with family will want to set aside some time to spend with family members. Figure 1-2 illustrates one student's time map for 1 week. Figure 1-3 provides an example of a blank time map.

Use a pencil when creating your time map, because your first estimates may not work. Adjust the schedule until it is more accurate for each activity, and do not forget to include at least a little time for the important people in your life and leisure time for yourself. Nothing but work and study may lead to burnout before the nursing program is completed. Enter all firm commitments, study times, time for completing assignments, and appointments in the calendar in this planner. Schedule class and study time on the time map first, working personal and social activities around them. Scheduling keeps your social time from interfering with sufficient study and sets you up for success in your nursing program. Using a calendar in Microsoft Outlook, Gmail, Yahoo!, or some other program is also advised. You will be sent reminders you've programmed for reviewing paper due dates and dates of upcoming tests.

SHARING HOUSEKEEPING TASKS

If you are living in a family situation, you need to delegate some tasks that were formerly yours to others in your household so that you can study the number of hours required for success in a nursing program. Your partner, if you have one, can help with household chores, run errands, and help with some of the tasks of childrearing. If adolescents are competent drivers, they can run errands and pick up and deliver smaller children for school or activities. See further suggestions in Chapter 3.

WORK ADJUSTMENTS

Once you decide to begin a nursing program, check with your employer about the possibility of flexible hours to accommodate the need for extra study time before examinations and for hospital clinical rotation requirements. Many employers will adjust hours for nursing students. **To give yourself the best chance at success in the nursing program, try not to work more than 20 hours per week.** The recommendations of one college regarding work and number of units undertaken are as follows:

40 hours work	Take only 6 units
30 hours work	Take only 9 units
20 hours work	Take only 12 units
10 hours work	Take only 15 units
0 hours work	Take 18 units

Courtesy Allan Hancock College, Santa Maria, CA.

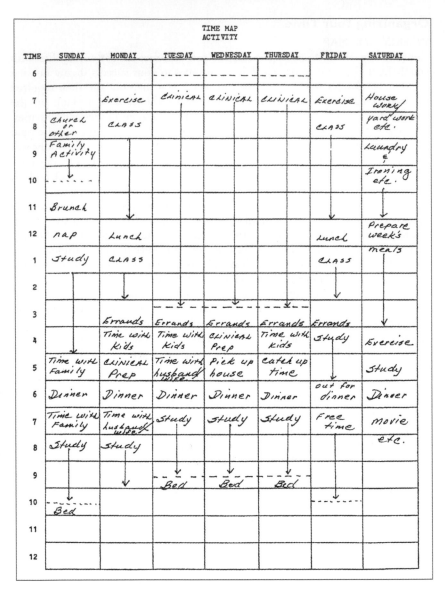

FIGURE 1-2 Sample time map.

If, after the first few months of the program, you find you have extra time when you could work and you are doing well academically, then you may be able to increase the number of work hours. Work hours may have to be adjusted again later in the program as courses become more demanding. If your employer is not able to adjust your schedule, you may wish to find a job working as a technician or as a patient care assistant in the local hospital during your training period. Many hospitals offer tuition reimbursement and flexible schedules for nursing students. Some hospitals have scholarship funds available for employees as well.

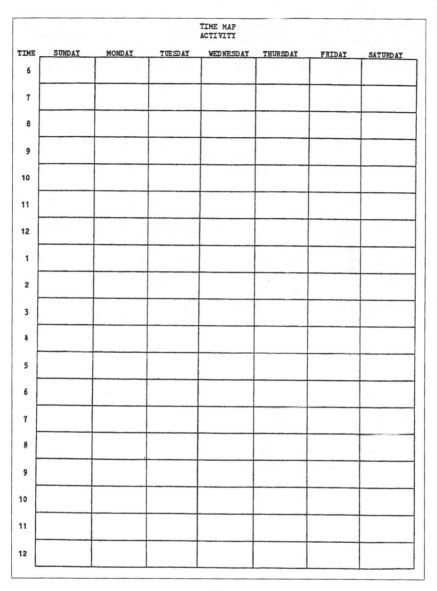

FIGURE I-3 Blank time map.

Another temporary or part-time job is as a student assistant on campus. Most colleges have a part-time work program available for students, including department "gofers," part-time secretaries or receptionists, laboratory helpers, classroom aides, library helpers, and similar positions. These positions are limited and are awarded to the quickest applicants.

A third possibility for part-time employment may be available for those who have a previous college degree or who excel in certain subjects such as mathematics, English, or science. A tutor in the college learning or tutoring center can earn

$9.00 or more per hour. The financial aid officer can provide information about grants and loans available and may also have scholarship information. The counseling center can assist you in your search for scholarship funds, as can both the school and local community librarians. Whatever your work schedule, enter your work hours in your calendar each week.

Study Skills

The study of nursing requires a great deal of reading. If you doubt your reading efficiency, contact your counselor or academic advisor and arrange to have your reading skills evaluated. Once the evaluation is done and any problem areas identified, methods by which your reading efficiency can be improved will be suggested. The few hours spent learning how to read more efficiently can save you study time in the future. Many schools offer a college learning skills course, and some institutions target sections specifically to health occupation students. Such a class, which is usually only 1 credit hour, can be a great tool for success in the nursing program.

Students in most nursing programs are expected to be proficient in how to access online materials and to use common software such as word processing and PowerPoint programs. Many schools are using eBooks for textbooks and are requiring the use of a laptop or iPad-type computer. Smart pens are available for taking notes and then transferring them to the computer for saving or printing. The pens are capable of recording audio lectures and then transferring the files to the computer as well.

Well-written professional nursing journal articles are invaluable resources. A bibliography or reference list for such articles is often included in your textbooks, the course outline or course syllabus. Check your college library's list of available journals in print or online (see Chapter 6). Ask the librarian to help if you are unfamiliar with accessing computerized databases. **Subscribing immediately to at least one of the major professional nursing journals when you enter nursing school is a time-saving idea.** Reading a journal each month will add considerably to your knowledge base in nursing. *Nursing 2015*, *Nursing Made Incredibly Easy*, and the *American Journal of Nursing* are three journals most useful to nursing students. *Imprint* is the National Student Nurses Association (NSNA) journal and has articles that are directed particularly to students rather than practicing nurses.

Various websites have very helpful study aids such as flash card programs for learning drug names. (See Chapter 6.)

LEARNING STYLES

Evaluating how you learn best is also helpful. Some people are visual learners, others are auditory learners, and some are tactile or kinesthetic learners, who learn best by doing. Most students have a predominant learning mode but use at least one of the other modes. The student learning center or counseling center, or the online tests listed in Chapter 6 can direct you in ways to evaluate your own learning style so that you can structure your studying around the best mode for you. If you are a visual learner, reading texts and articles and watching visual presentations via the computer or video are the best ways to spend your study time. If you are an auditory learner, then recording lectures, listening to supplementary CDs or MP3 lecture files, which are available at some schools, and perhaps reading and recording your texts for future listening are the best ways to study. A tactile learner needs to spend extra time in the skill and simulation lab or at home practicing the skills step by step, preferably with a peer watching. Computer-based instruction may also assist this type of learner by allowing some tactile interaction during the lesson. The actual performance of skills and patient care in the clinical setting is the other major mode of learning available for a tactile learner. Elsevier's *Virtual Clinical Excursions*, which are designed to complement your textbooks and incorporate visual, auditory, and kinesthetic learning, are available at your college bookstore or online from Elsevier Inc.

TEXTBOOKS

Buy your required textbooks immediately in eBook or paper form, and put your name in any paper text. When studying, remember to check each possible text that might contain information required for the next day's lecture topics. Text information frequently changes in the health occupation field; therefore, relying on a friend's old textbooks is not a good idea. The required textbooks are essential to your success. If you cannot afford a textbook right now, visit the library to determine whether a copy is "on reserve." Read the library copy and make buying your own textbook a top priority.

Reading

You will absorb more from your reading if you find a quiet place with few distractions. If you must read with activity going on around you, consider masking the noise and distraction by using a pair of foam earplugs (available at pharmacies) or headphones with soft music playing. Some students who are parents have found that it is best for them to go to bed at the same time as their children, get up in the middle of the night for a few hours to read and study, and then sleep a few more hours before the beginning of the day.

Read in an organized, consistent manner. **Look up unfamiliar words** in the glossary of the text or a dictionary as you encounter them, and jot down their meanings. The SQ4R study method (Box 1-3) is a popular plan for tackling reading and study assignments. Try it; if it does not suit your needs, check your college library and bookstore for study books containing other methods.

Reading is the key to establishing the base of knowledge needed to function as a nurse. If you can find time to read full chapters rather than just a few pages about a particular disease or problem, you will remember the information more easily and develop a fuller understanding of the body systems, how homeostasis is affected by diseases, and why particular nursing interventions are effective in a particular instance. From the beginning of nursing school, studying this way tends to make reading assignments less lengthy and makes the upper-level courses much easier, because you will already have read much of the material to be covered.

Nursing textbooks are large and heavy. If you have time to study at work, consider an e-reader (e.g., Kindle, iPad, Nook). Textbook companies have developed interactive texts for online use. If this is not an option, consider tearing out individual chapters in your paper textbook to take to work with you. Heavy books are difficult to carry, but single chapters are easily portable. (This may sound like heresy when you have been taught not to damage a book, but it is a practical solution.) Be certain to keep the chapters neatly filed for future review.

Students who have difficulty reading because of dyslexia or visual problems should contact the Braille Institute Library Services (1-800-272-4553; 741 North

BOX 1-3

SQ4R Study Method

S Survey   **R** Read   **R** Record (Write)
Q Question   **R** Recite   **R** Review

Survey	Look over the chapter. Read all the headings, captions under photographs, and all illustrations, charts, and graphs, plus the summary or last paragraph. This survey provides the core ideas in the chapter.
Question	Make a question out of each heading. Doing so arouses curiosity, focuses on the content, and brings to mind information you already know.
Read	Begin actively reading for an answer to the question. Read only one section and be certain you have answered the question before continuing. Highlight or underline the important points as you find them.
Recite	After finishing each section, look away from the book and, using your own words, recite the answer to your question. If you can do this, you know what is in the book. If you cannot, you need to reread the section and consider. Continue in this manner through the entire reading assignment. Write study notes for your objectives as you finish each section by either writing an answer to the objective or by making an outline for the items listed in the content column of the syllabus.
Record (write)	Record the information in some fashion. Use a highlighter to mark directly on the specific information in the text, take notes, or use a combination of the two. It is important to read and understand the material first and then go back and record.
Review	When you have finished the assignment for the next lecture session, review your notes to understand the points and their relationships to one another. Check your memory by trying to answer each objective in the syllabus without looking at your notes.

Vermont Avenue, Los Angeles, CA 90029). Students who qualify can receive recordings of various nursing textbooks as well as a tape or CD player to use with them.

Using Ancillary Materials

Check out web pages designated for your textbooks or the CDs packaged with them, which usually contain a significant amount of good information. They may include extras that would not fit into the text chapters, animations for various concepts or processes, audio pronunciation files, links to useful resources, and many other features. Checking for updates on the textbook's accompanying website is a good idea.

A helpful study guide or workbook may be available for your nursing text. If study guides are not *required*, check your bookstore or the Internet to see whether any are available for your texts. Many students find such resources useful learning tools.

Taking Notes

Two types of notes should be taken: (1) preparatory notes taken before class and (2) class notes taken during a lecture or lab, which build on your preparatory notes. Preparation before class greatly enhances learning, because the material covered in class is not being encountered for the first time. **Repetition is essential to the retention of information.** Some eBook texts are interactive online, through Pageburst or similar software. The software allows you to add notes as you read, highlight material, and note questions. Familiarity with the topics to be covered in class allows you to follow the instructor's presentation by listening actively and adding to notes as needed. (When you attempt to take extensive notes during class, you might miss much of what the instructor is saying.)

Consult the course outline or syllabus to identify material that will be covered during each class. First, read the required selection in your textbook, underlining or highlighting key concepts in the text, tables, charts, and illustrations. Then create preparatory study notes by outlining the material covered in required reading or by writing out concise answers to the lecture or chapter objectives. When writing study notes, use an organizational method that allows for the addition of information during the lecture. As study notes are enhanced during the lecture, they become class notes.

Some instructors may provide PowerPoint slides or other outlines for students to download and bring to class. This is a handy way to take organized notes in class. Two examples are offered in Figure 1-4. Review each set of revised notes as soon as possible after class, review all notes for the week every weekend, and review all notes for material to be covered on an examination in the few days preceding the test.

Considering what would make a good examination question out of this material is also helpful. What questions would you ask if you were the instructor? Jot down your ideas. After the examination on this material, go back to see how many of these questions were on the test. While preparing for class, jot down any points that are unclear, but wait until the end of class to ask the questions, because the instructor will likely answer them or clarify the topic during class time.

Along with the required readings, the syllabus may also list other learning resources, such as related periodical articles from professional nursing journals, media presentations, and computer learning modules. Whenever material is difficult to understand or unclear, using one or two of these other resources can greatly improve comprehension and retention of the material.

Recording Lectures

Some schools provide PowerPoint with voice-over lectures on the school intranet. These are to be used before class time. The class time then provides other types of learning activities facilitated by the instructor. This is termed a "flipped classroom" method of teaching. Some schools still use the traditional lecture method for class time. If you have difficulty following a particular instructor's presentation or simply do not "get" all the information in a lecture, you may want to use an audio or video recorder during class (after obtaining the instructor's permission). It has often been said that the average student hears only 30% of what is said during a class period. Taking the time to listen to or watch the recordings and adding to your study notes as appropriate are necessary for the success of this type of study. You also can play audio recordings in the car when traveling to and from

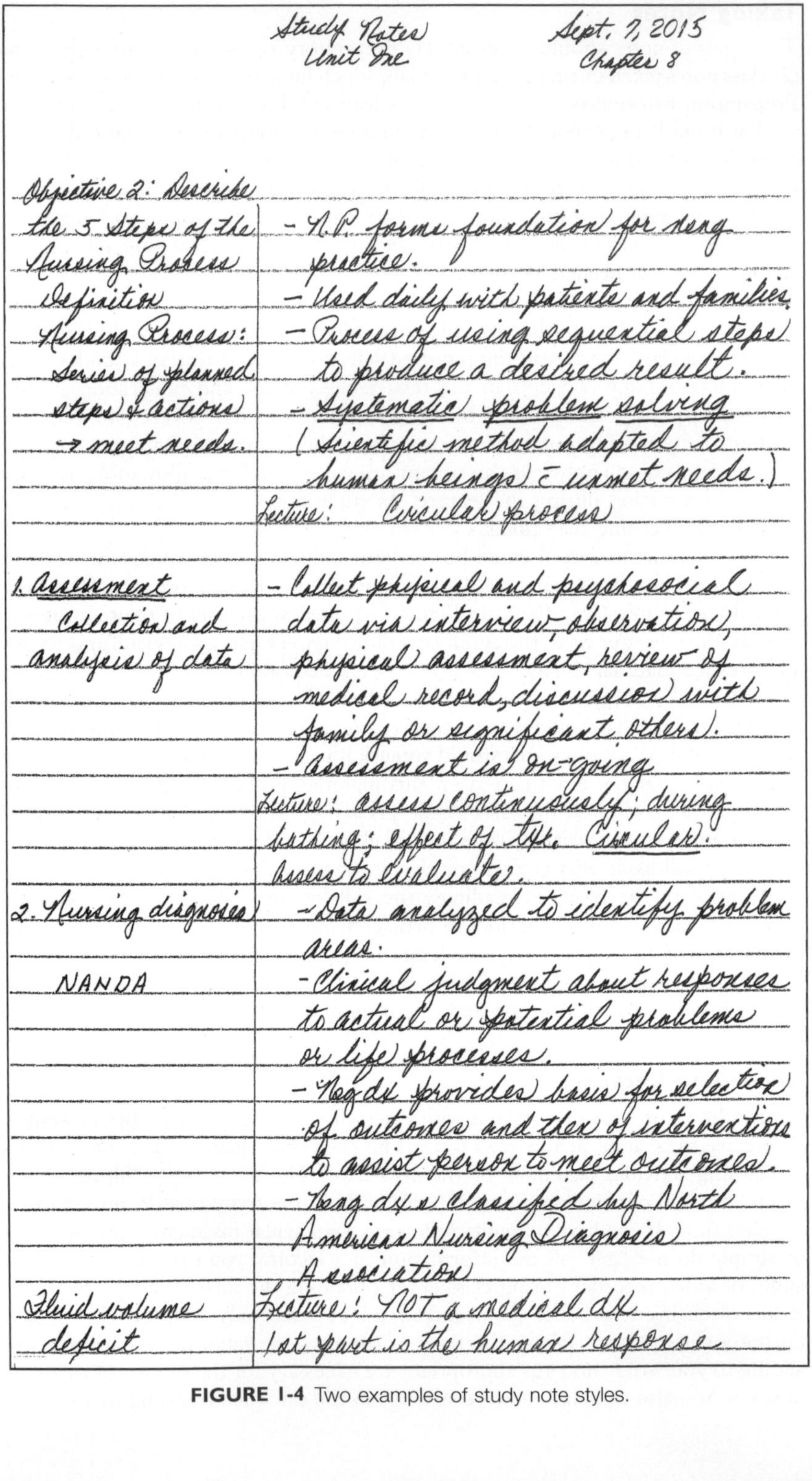

Study Notes   *Sept. 7, 2015*
Unit One   *Chapter 8*

Objective 2: Describe the 5 Steps of the Nursing Process	– N.P. forms foundation for nsng. practice.
Definition	– Used daily with patients and families.
Nursing Process: Series of planned steps & actions → meet needs.	– Process of using sequential steps to produce a desired result. – Systematic *problem solving* (Scientific method adapted to human beings c̄ unmet needs.) Lecture: Circular process
1. Assessment Collection and analysis of data	– Collect physical and psychosocial data via interview, observation, physical assessment, review of medical record, discussion with family or significant others). – Assessment is on-going Lecture: assess continuously; during bathing; effect of tx. Circular. Assess to evaluate.
2. Nursing diagnoses NANDA	– Data analyzed to identify problem areas. – Clinical judgment about responses to actual or potential problems or life processes. – Nsg dx provides basis for selection of outcomes and then of interventions to assist person to meet outcomes. – Nsg dx is classified by North American Nursing Diagnosis Association
Fluid volume deficit	Lecture: NOT a medical dx. 1st part is the human response.

FIGURE 1-4 Two examples of study note styles.

Study Notes — Sept. 8, 2015
Chapter 8

Obj. 2   Describe the 5 steps of the nursing process

I. Nursing process	Lecture:
A. Foundation of practice	Circular, systematic
B. Used daily	process similar to
C. Sequential steps to-	scientific method.
ward desired result	Use with every patient.
D. systematic problem	Core of professional
solving	nursing. Methodical
	and orderly.
II. Assessment	Assessment is on-going.
A. Physical & psychosocial	Constantly assess - during
data gathered	both & txs. Response to
1) patient	meds. Assess in order to
2) chart	evaluate. Use all senses.
3) family / S.O.	History taking via inter-
B. Analysis of data	view. Physical assessment
III. Nursing diagnosis	Data analyzed to find
A. Identify human	problem areas. Requires
response	Clinical judgment.
B. Related factors	North
C. Pertinent defining	American
characteristics	Nursing
D. Choose from NANDA	Diagnoses
list	Association
	Not a medical dx.
	Basis for choosing
	interventions to alleviate
	human response.

FIGURE 1-4, cont'd

school and work or while preparing meals, doing yard work, ironing, or performing other household chores that lend themselves to listening while doing.

Strengthening Computer Skills

Honing your computer skills will make you a more efficient and better organized student and nurse. You likely will be expected to use a unit computer to enter data about patient care when working or participating in clinical rotations and a word processing program such as Microsoft Word to create nursing care plans and written assignments. As you progress through your nursing courses, creating nursing care plans electronically can save a lot of repetitious writing. With files of saved care plans, you can cut and paste, individualizing the new plan for a particular patient.

Microsoft Excel is also a valuable program to learn and is used in almost any job. Microsoft PowerPoint will most likely be needed by students asked to make class presentations. This presentation software is used throughout the business world. E-mail is valuable for contacting fellow students and instructors and is also a useful way for a busy nursing student to stay in touch with friends. Skype or Face-Time can be used to work from home with other students.

The Internet is a wonderful source for information on medical and nursing topics, including patient teaching. Blogs, message boards, and e-mail lists covering topics specific to nurses or nursing students can help you get answers to questions and provide a support group. You will be asked to do research, and the Internet has a wealth of information (and misinformation). Knowing how to evaluate the sites and information you find is essential (Box 1-4).

Joining a Study Group

Depending on your learning style, you may find that joining a study group helps you better prepare for tests. The advantage of being in a study group is that you receive the benefit of the other members' viewpoints on topics and what is most important in the material to be covered on a test. Some study groups divide up

---

BOX 1-4

Evaluating a Web Page

- Who wrote the page? What are the person's qualifications and associations? Can you contact him or her?
- What institution publishes this page? Check the domain of the document in the URL. Preferred domains are *.edu, .gov, .org,* and *.net.*
- When was the web page produced? Is it current and timely? Has it been updated since it was written?
- Is the information cited authentic? Can you verify it with other sources?
- What is the purpose of the web page?
- What is the point of view? What opinions are expressed by the author? Is bias evident? If so, what is it?
- Is the web page written objectively?
- Could the web page be a spoof or ironic?
- Are questions or reservations you have about the web page answered or satisfied?
- How up to date are the links (if they are provided)?

the objectives of a unit, and each member prepares the answers to a certain number of the objectives. This method works well if each member does a thorough job. However, some students cannot simply read and memorize material; they retain the information better if they write it out themselves. When looking for a study group, **remember that studying with people who are more knowledgeable than you and earning as good or better grades is to your advantage.**

When working with a study group, complete the reading and prepare for a discussion before you meet. Discussing the material will round out your knowledge of the subject, and hearing about it again will reinforce it in your memory.

Obtaining Tutoring

Check with the tutoring center, learning center, learning resources center, or college handbook to see whether tutoring service is available. Tutoring services are often free to students and are provided by a higher-level student who has earned a high grade point average. Sometimes tutoring is available on a fee-for-service basis. The main point is to seek help as soon as you determine that you could use it.

Taking an Online Course

When considering an online course, ask yourself whether you are a self-motivator and highly disciplined about schoolwork. Without face-to-face contact with an instructor, you will need to take the initiative in obtaining assignments, requesting clarification when questions arise, and completing required work. Before signing up for an online course, explore the course description and requirements, be certain that the computer you will use meets the minimum specifications and that you have the required software installed, and make sure the course will meet your needs (such as credit toward graduation, prerequisite credit for another course you will take later, or other requirements). If the class is offered by a different college from the one you are attending, be certain the credit will be transferable. Determine whether your level of computer competence is sufficient to get you through the course (Box 1-5).

Once you are enrolled, determine the instructor's expectations. If they are not clear, e-mail the instructor and ask for the specific expectations. Consider the expectations and how your own strengths fit with what is expected. Consider the challenges you will face in the course. Do you have the technical skills you will need? Become familiar with the software platform (e.g., Blackboard, WebCT, E-College, etc.) through which the online course will be offered. If you are unfamiliar with the platform, work through the tutorial for it. If you have doubts about your academic research or computer skills, check with your librarian or the computer lab personnel. They can recommend materials and tutorials that may be helpful.

Time management is extremely important when you engage in distance learning. If the instructor sets virtual office hours, plan your study time around them to ensure that he or she will be available to answer questions quickly if they arise. If specific times for communication with fellow students or with the instructor are set, be online and available. Write these times into your daily time map.

Many online classes are organized into a series of modules. Set up files for each module, and keep everything together that pertains to each module. This method of organization will help you have everything ready when you work on a particular module. Accordion files are great for papers related to the module.

BOX 1-5

Computer Competency Checklist for Nursing Classes

You should know how to use the following software:

- Operating system (e.g., Microsoft Windows)
- Word processing program (e.g., Microsoft Word)
- Presentation program (e.g., Microsoft PowerPoint)
- Spreadsheet program (e.g., Microsoft Excel)
- Database (e.g., Microsoft Access)

You should be able to:

- Gain access to an Internet service or service provider, preferably high speed.
- Enable a firewall.
- Use a virus protection program.
- Install software programs.
- Install plug-ins.
- Save a file of your work to your hard drive and a CD or flash drive.
- Download and save files.
- Copy, cut, and paste sections of text within a document and between documents.
- Use an Internet search engine.
- Search for information and articles on a given subject.
- Reload a page in a Web browser.
- Clear the cache or temporary Internet files in a Web browser.

For accessing and handling e-mail, you should be able to:

- Set up an e-mail account with an Internet provider.
- Send, receive, and open e-mail messages.
- Open e-mail attachments.
- Reply to e-mail messages.
- Print e-mail messages.
- Save e-mail messages to folders.
- Attach files to e-mail messages.
- Delete e-mail messages.

Be aware that Internet searches can be very time consuming. Schedule enough time to conduct your research, and start well ahead of the paper or project due date. Check the class bulletin board daily for postings from faculty or students.

Note that communication within an online course is slower than that in the classroom. A delay may occur often between sending an e-mail question to the instructor and receiving an answer. When you do not understand something about an assignment or a reading, immediately seek clarification from the instructor. Be patient when waiting for an answer; do not send repeat e-mails with the same questions.

Often an online course will require you to work as part of a group on a project. Try to balance your interaction so that you do not end up doing more than your share of the project. Keep communication open and timely among the group members so that progress on each part of the project will be evident. Because your grade depends on all members of the group finishing their portions, plan some extra time to help pick up the slack if someone does not come through with his or her part of the work.

Taking online classes can be beneficial because they are more time flexible than on-campus classes. You alone are responsible for scheduling when you will go online to do your class work. Some degree programs can be accomplished entirely by taking online courses (see Chapter 4).

Doing Your Best on Tests

It is a good idea at the beginning of each week to scan your calendar for the next test date. The best way to decrease test anxiety is to study the material sufficiently and get a good night's sleep before the examination. Last-minute cramming does not work for most people. **Cell phones are not allowed in testing areas at most schools.** Because the National Council Licensure Examination (NCLEX) is a timed exam, nursing school tests have a time limit in which to complete answering the test questions. Testing may be done via computer in a designated computer room.

PREPARATION

When organizing to study specifically for an examination, review the instructor's designation of the material to be covered on this particular test. Conduct this review at least 1 week before the test. Gather revised preparatory notes, and rewrite the data that you feel are most important (and likely to be included on the test) in a concise form. Include material from special sources, such as required presentations or articles. Review your concise test notes each night.

Divide the material into the same number of parts as number of days before the test, and systematically review your full notes at least once more. If time permits, you can go back and review what you have highlighted in your texts as well. If you belong to a study group, meet on the day before the examination and question one another on the objectives and what the group believes is the most important material as well as the material an instructor will most likely include in the examination. When preparing for an exam, be certain you know which type of testing will be used (computer or paper). Exams may use only generic drug names in questions as that is how the NCLEX exam questions are written. Nursing diagnoses are not used on the NCLEX exam.

Day before the examination. Review the syllabus or course outline of the material to be covered on the test. Read the content column, as well as the objectives, and review anything you cannot immediately recall. Pay close attention to the vocabulary and terms.

Night before the examination. Get at least 7 hours of sleep. Eat a normal meal before going to school. If the test is late in the morning, take a high-power snack with you to eat 20 minutes before the examination. The brain works best when it has the glucose necessary for cellular function. Stay away from other nervous students before the test. Stop reviewing at least 30 minutes before the test. Take a walk, go to the library and read a magazine, listen to music, or do something else that is relaxing. Go to the test room a few minutes before class time so that you are not rushed in settling down in your seat. Tune out what others are saying. Crowd tension is contagious, so stay away from it.

During the examination

Paper tests. You can enhance your chance of success during a test. The following are several suggestions for taking tests on paper:

- Note the number of questions and the total time allotted for the test to calculate the times at which you should be halfway and three-quarters finished with the test. Allow 5 to 10 minutes to check your work and your answer sheet. Look at the clock only every 10 minutes or so.
- Carefully read the preliminary instructions and check the whiteboard or screen at the front of the room for any changes or correction of printing errors.
- Calm yourself by closing your eyes, putting down your pencil, and relaxing. Deep-breathe for a few minutes (or as needed, if you feel especially tense) to relax your body and to relieve tension.
- If you are allowed to write on the test booklet, underline all pertinent data and circle key words in the question.
- Cover the answer options before reading the question on multiple choice tests. Read the question and think about what the answer(s) should be; then see whether such an answer is among the choices.
- For questions in which you need to "select all that apply," cover the answers while looking at the question stem and think about what fits. Then look at each of the choices and circle the number or letter of each choice that correctly fits with the question. For fill-in-the-blank exercises, choose the word or words that immediately come to mind. Some questions will ask you to identify a spot on an anatomic model where you would do something or where something occurs. Locate the landmarks on the model carefully before indicating the correct spot.
- Eliminate wrong choices by marking through the letters or numbers of those choices.
- After choosing an answer, go back and reread the question stem along with your chosen answer. Does it fit correctly? The choice that grammatically fits the stem and contains the correct information is the best choice.
- Do not read too much into the question or worry that it is a "trick." If you have nursing experience, ask yourself how a classmate who is inexperienced would answer this question from only the information provided in the textbooks or given in the lectures.
- If you do not understand the question or a word within the question, raise your hand and ask the instructor for clarification.
- Avoid choosing answers that use words such as *always, never, must, all*, and *none*. If you are confused about the question, read the choices, label them *true* or *false*, and choose the answer that is the odd one out (i.e., the one false one or the one true one). When a question is framed in the negative, such as "When assessing for pain, you should *not* ... ," the false option is the correct choice.
- Do not fret over any one question for too long. If you are having trouble, skip the question and go back to it when you have finished answering the other questions.
- If using a paper Scantron sheet, keep track of the correlating test question number. When you skip a question, be careful to also skip the corresponding space on the Scantron sheet.
- Check your Scantron sheet to ensure that every line has only one mark; two marks on any one line would throw all the remaining answers off track from the correct question numbers.

- Choose the *best* answer for questions asking for a single answer. More than one answer may be correct, but one answer may contain more information or more important information than another answer.
- When you are unsure, jot down what you know about the topic in the margin, or on permitted scratch paper, without looking at the answers. Then look at the answers and follow your best instinct.
- **Never erase and change an answer on a Scantron sheet** unless you have read the question or the answer incorrectly or remember a specific piece of information that has a bearing on the question. If you realize that you missed questions on previous tests because you erased and changed answers, cut the eraser off the end of the pencil you take to the examination. If you find you have read a question wrong and really need to erase, raise your hand and ask the instructor for an eraser. This technique has helped numerous students raise their test grades considerably.
- At the end of the test, reread the questions, making certain you understood each one correctly. Verify that the answer sheet is marked in the right location for each answer.

Computer-based tests. Many of these suggestions also are useful for tests administered via computer. In addition to these tips, it is wise to practice on the type of computer on which the test will be given. Maintaining focus without becoming distracted by people entering and leaving the room can be a challenge. Monitoring your time is very important. Most computer tests do not penalize you for guessing at an answer. With computer testing, usually you will not be able to skip questions and go back to answer them later. You will not be able to change an answer once you have progressed to the next question. Ask whether you will be allowed scratch paper in the computer testing room. Be certain you know the times the test is available for you to take in the testing location.

- When entering the test, click the link only once. It may take a while to load.
- Do not use the "back" button.
- Do not double click on an answer. A second click may be read as a second attempt to answer and may block further access to the test.
- Do not click "Submit," "Next," or "Save" more than once for each question.
- Do click on a blank area when using a mouse with a scroll wheel so that you don't accidentally change an answer when scrolling.
- Answer all the questions.
- If possible, review all your answers before you click "Submit" to enter your test answers at the end of the test. Click "Submit" only once.
- If the test is timed, you may be given a 1-minute warning before time is up. Be certain to click "Submit" before the time is up.

ALTERNATE-FORMAT QUESTIONS
You may find that questions on your examinations are not always multiple choice, in which a single option of four given is correct, and many are patterned after the types used on the NCLEX. Alternate-format questions include the following types; correct answers are given.

Multiple response. A patient is prescribed a low-fat diet. In counseling him or her about food choices, you would tell him or her to avoid *(select all that apply)*:

1. Butter
2. Barbecued ribs
3. Grilled salmon
4. Caesar salad
5. Hamburgers
6. Whole milk
Answer: 1, 2, 5, 6

Illustration/graphic. The nurse is performing a physical examination on a patient. When listening to the heart, the nurse would place the stethoscope over the apex to count the apical pulse. Indicate on the diagram the location of the apex of the heart. (Place the cursor over the correct area and click.)

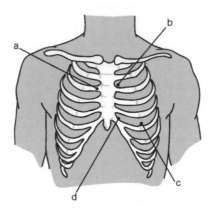

Answer: C

Prioritization/sequencing. When catheterizing a female patient, the nurse would use sterile technique. Place the steps of the catheterization procedure in the correct sequence.

1. Lubricate the catheter.
2. Don sterile gloves.
3. Cleanse the meatus.
4. Drape the genital area.
5. Locate the urinary meatus.
6. Insert the catheter.
Answer: 5, 4, 2, 3, 1, 6

Completion/fill-in-the-blank. A patient has an intravenous (IV) infusion ordered of D_5 ½ NS 1000 mL at 100 mL/hr. If the IV tubing will deliver 15 drops per mL, the IV should be set to deliver _____ drops per minute.
Answer: 25

Chart/exhibition. A patient had surgery yesterday with bleeding at the surgical site. Serial laboratory hemoglobin and hematocrit values have been measured as follows:

	1600	2200	0800	1400
Hemoglobin	10.8 mg/dL	10.2 mg/dL	10.2 mg/dL	10.4 mg/dL
Hematocrit	28%	26%	26%	27%

Assessment of the data reveals that:

1. Slow bleeding may be occurring.
2. Considerable blood loss occurred.
3. Red blood cell count has stabilized.
4. Red blood cell count shows hemodilution.

Answer: 3

Other question types. Other question types include true-false (mark true or false), short answer (write a brief answer), and matching (you are asked to choose the correct companions from column 2 that correlate with statements or items in column 1). NCLEX questions are also written in the traditional multiple-choice format (one correct answer from a choice of four).

ESSAY EXAMINATIONS

- Divide the total testing time by the number of questions to be completed.
- Quickly outline the content of your answer before you begin writing.
- Answer the questions you know best first; doing so will help build your confidence.
- If you do not think you know the answer, take a little time to jot down everything you know about the topic and then try to formulate an answer.
- If you have absolutely no clue as to the answer to a question, try to think of something creative to write. Sometimes an instructor will give you a few points for creativity. Anything is better than a blank space on an essay examination.
- Reread each question and the answer you have written, making certain that it actually answers the question asked.
- Be certain your handwriting is legible.
- Pay attention to correct grammar, punctuation, and spelling.

ACADEMIC HONESTY

Most colleges have an honesty policy or code, and nursing as a profession expects its members to be honest and ethical. Although learning may involve group activities, you must write papers or care plans alone and submit your own work. Colleges have software programs to detect plagiarism (work done by another but submitted as one's own). Cheating on tests—including copying from another's test paper or computer screen, acquiring answers from or giving answers to another person by any means, discussing questions or topics from a test with another student yet to take the exams, and sneaking information into the testing area in any form—is often a cause for dismissal from a nursing program. Cheating does not prepare the student to pass the NCLEX.

If you think that an assignment is meant to be a group project and allows collaboration with others, verify that with the instructor. If you are writing a research paper, make sure you understand how to reference sources. Not giving credit to information sources is considered plagiarism. Cheating is a serious matter in nursing education because you must thoroughly know the information being taught to become a safe nurse. Once you become a registered or practical nurse, the lives of your patients are in your hands. **A mistake can mean serious injury or death.**

A saying in the human resources field is, "Past practice predicts future performance." If you cheat as a student, the prediction is that you may continue to do so as a nurse. Nurses have the privilege and responsibility of caring for patients when they are most vulnerable, and ethical practice is at the heart of nursing. Patients trust nurses and count on them to do what is in the best interest of the patient. Be worthy of that trust.

TROUBLESHOOTING EXAMINATION PERFORMANCE

If you are not achieving the scores you would like or think you deserve, review the following questions to find ways in which you might improve your chance to score higher:

- How many hours per week are you spending in quality, uninterrupted study time?
- How well can you concentrate during each segment of your study time? Are you too tired to concentrate?
- How many hours are you working? How many credit hours are you taking? Do you have enough hours in the week to study adequately?
- Are you doing your reading before class? Are you reading whole chapters?
- Are you reading in each pertinent textbook (fundamentals of nursing, medical–surgical nursing, pediatric nursing, obstetric nursing, nutrition, psychiatric nursing, and pharmacology, among others)?
- How do you begin a unit of study? Do you review the pertinent anatomy and physiology before beginning the text readings if you do not remember it?
- Do you study the objectives in the syllabus as you go, including the topics in the content column?
- Are you utilizing other assigned activities before class?
- Do you take study notes after you have first read the material but before the lecture in a format that allows you to add lecture notes to your study notes?
- Do you use a voice recorder in class? Do you review the recordings?
- Do you experience greater than normal test anxiety? Have you worked with a counselor for this anxiety? Have you regularly practiced suggested relaxation and confidence-building techniques?
- Do you review each day's lecture notes that night?
- Are you using effective test-taking techniques, as follows:
  - Becoming comfortable with the computer-type testing before the exam?
  - Underlining key words in the stem and choices (for paper tests)?
  - Eliminating wrong choices?
  - Checking to ensure that your chosen answer fits with the question stem and that it answers the question asked?
  - Using test time evenly?
  - Refraining from frequently erasing and changing answers?

- Do you have a regular study group or study partner? Are the others in the group doing well? (If not, study with someone who is!)
- Are you relying on reading in a review book to get you through instead of reading your texts?
- Are you relying on reading in a review book before tests instead of studying your own notes?

If you identify your problem areas and remedy them, your test scores will improve. Students often believe that they study a lot, but they study at home with constant interruptions to their concentration. Going to the neighborhood library to study is one option. Organizing to study during the day when roommates, partners, and children are out of the house, and then doing chores, shopping, laundry, and errands at night, is another alternative.

Problems at school should be remedied as soon as they are identified. Many students believe their school experiences will improve without taking any initiative to make certain that they do. Too often, students wait until they are in serious trouble with poor grades before changing their study habits or the number of hours they work. You have invested a lot in your education; guard that investment by giving yourself the best chance for success.

A psychological technique used to boost your test-taking confidence is to look into a mirror whenever you pass one and say out loud, "I know the material, and I'll do well on the test." Try it; many students have found that it works because it reduces "test anxiety."

Taking the National Council Licensure Examination

During your final semester, you will receive information from your instructors on the mechanics of signing up to take the NCLEX, which is taken on a computer at a designated testing site. After you graduate from your nursing program and have met the educational requirements for licensure, your school will notify the state board of nursing that you have completed the required courses for licensure. You must submit an application for licensure to the state board of nursing, and then you will receive a ticket that allows you to sit for the NCLEX-RN or NCLEX-PN, depending on which type of program you have completed. The examinations are offered at sites across the United States. If you do not pass the test on the first attempt, you must wait 45 to 90 days (depending on the state you are in) before retaking it. The examination may be taken in any state, but licensure will be issued by the state in which you reside. Visit *www.ncsbn.com* to view the test plan, a variety of resources to help you prepare for the examination, and a list of states that have a reciprocity compact agreement for licensure (in which license is obtained in one state but education and passing the exam make one eligible to obtain a license in another state).

Obtaining Licensure

After passing the NCLEX-PN or NCLEX-RN, you will receive a licensure ticket from the testing center. That ticket, along with the paperwork from your school documenting completion of the required courses and clinical hours, must be submitted along with the application for licensure to your state board of nurse examiners.

2 GETTING THE MOST FROM THE CLINICAL EXPERIENCE

■ APPROACHING THE CLINICAL EXPERIENCE

You may be assigned to various clinical facilities during the semester. Clinical locations include hospitals, long-term care facilities, home health agencies, community clinics, psychiatric outpatient clinics, day care centers, and school clinics. At some of these facilities you may be an observer rather than a care provider. Your instructor will clarify how you should prepare for the type of clinical facility to which you are assigned.

It is normal to be concerned and apprehensive about your first contact with a patient. Be assured that you will not be required to do more for the patient than your nursing course has prepared you to do. Remember that there is always a staff nurse assigned to the patient as well. It is usual for the student to prepare at school for the skills to be performed in the clinical setting and to be evaluated on critical skills by an instructor. Only then are you expected to apply your skills with real patients. Critical skills are those in which accuracy is of vital importance to the patient's treatment (e.g., taking vital signs) or those that are invasive and have a potential for injury to the patient (e.g., giving an injection, inserting a urinary catheter).

If you are entering the room to take vital signs, be certain you have all your equipment with you including appropriate documentation resources—paper, handheld electronic device, or in-room computer.

Most students fear hurting the patient. The best way to prevent harm is to be as prepared as possible for the clinical patient assignment and to refuse to perform tasks for which instruction and verification of the correct technique by an instructor have not yet occurred. Tell the nurse in charge of the patient that you may not perform the skill or care involved if you have not covered it in school.

Preparing for Clinical Patient Care

At some schools, instructors assign patients to the students; other schools require that each student choose patients for the clinical assignment. Either way, you will receive some pertinent information ahead of time. Before you see the patient, you will know the patient's diagnosis, what treatments are scheduled, any tests the patient may have that day, the names of the medications, and the patient's age and sex. Conduct a quick review of each patient's chart when obtaining your information (Table 2-1). In addition, ask to see the patient care card, Kardex plan, or electronic patient care sheets. These provide directions for everything the nurse should be doing for the patient. Look for the nursing care plan or the "problem" list in the chart; both will give you some ideas about the patient's nursing problems and actual nursing diagnoses. Before selecting your assignment, check with the nurse in charge to ensure that you know which patients other students have already selected.

TABLE 2-1   Quick Chart Review

Sheet	Information
Face sheet or electronic patient record (EMR) sheet	Marital status, age, insurance coverage, occupation, significant others, religion, location of home
Physician's order sheet	Tests ordered, medications, intravenous solutions, treatments to be done, code status (admitting day up to today)
Physician's history and physical (H & P)	Overview of total health status and summary of current and physical health problems; allergies
Physician's progress notes	Clues to future tests and orders; status of notes problems
Nursing admission assessment	Medications and supplements taken at home, allergies; height and weight; prosthetic devices such as hearing aids, glasses, or contact lenses; previous health problems and hospitalizations; previous surgery; and so forth
Laboratory reports	Tests that have been completed, results, and any abnormal values
Other test results	Findings that are abnormal (read the conclusions); pathology reports tell whether patient has cancer
Medication administration record (MAR)	Medications ordered; how often patient is taking as-needed (PRN) medications and what they are
Consultations	Conclusions of other members of the health care team
Nurse's notes	Care given for previous 24 hours; problems encountered; changes in plan of care; visitors; psychological outlook
Flow sheets and EMR	Vital signs, intake and output, intravenous fluids, blood administered, neurological signs and changes, and so forth
Nursing care plan, collaborative care plan, care pathway, or "needs" list	Lists the problems or nursing diagnoses, with goals and care interventions to be done
Operative report	Conclusion tells what was done; abnormalities found and problems encountered; amount of blood loss

Preparing for clinical patient care involves reading about the disease process or problem and noting the following:

- Causes and contributing (etiologic) factors
- Usual signs and symptoms of the disorder
- Common medical treatment for the disorder, including medications
- Common nursing problems or nursing diagnoses the patient is likely to have
- Expected outcomes
- Psychosocial ramifications

If you are not assigned a specific patient before your clinical experience, find out which unit you will be assigned to and determine the types of patients usually cared for on that unit. Then read about those types of patients. For example, if you are assigned to an orthopedic unit, you should read about fractures, traction, back problems, and hip and knee replacements. When assigned to a general surgical unit, review preoperative and postoperative care, dressing changes, nasogastric suction, and care of wound suction devices and catheters, among others. Your textbooks will give you clues about the information you will need for the type of hospital unit in which you will be working. An Internet search can usually provide information on the disease or condition a patient has and the appropriate care. Search by subject or enter a medical site such as those listed in Chapter 6. If you do not have your own computer or a smartphone, use one available at your school or the public library.

Reviewing Skills for Patient Care

Review information about the treatments to be provided, such as dressing changes, maintaining traction, hot or cold applications, and intravenous (IV) therapy. You should review each treatment even if it is not a task you are capable of doing. Clinical learning takes place when you are prepared and observe an experienced nurse perform the skill. Of course, as each nursing course progresses, you will be prepared to perform more of the skills. Instructors generally require that the student review a skill just before performing it in the clinical area.

When on the nursing unit, you can look up the skill or treatment in the procedure manual kept on the floor or in the computer. Each nursing unit should have a manual available to staff that provides the specific steps and protocol for performing each nursing procedure. To be within safe, legal boundaries, each nurse should perform the designated procedure in the manner described. It is up to the student to seek experience in performing skills. Choose patients for your assignment who require some skills you can perform. During the report, mention that when your assigned work is done, you would like to perform other tasks for which you are prepared. Be specific about what you are looking for such as injections, catheterizations, or IV therapy experience.

Looking Up Medications

From clinical day 1, you should look up each medication your assigned patients are receiving. Learn the generic as well as the most common brand name. Although students do not usually administer medications during the first weeks of the first nursing course, the best way to learn about the thousands of medications in use is to attach a patient situation to each. Even if you are not giving the medication, you will be expected to watch for possible side effects of various drugs. **You are legally liable if you cause harm to a patient from a medication error you committed.**

DRUG TEXT APP OR HANDBOOK

If you have a pharmacology text, look up and review each patient's medication(s). If you do not have such a text, you may wish to purchase a drug reference written especially for nurses or an application (app) for your smartphone or tablet. Many such books are available on the market, and your school bookstore probably stocks a variety of handbooks. Information you want includes the following:

- Classification of the drug (e.g., antibiotic, antihypertensive)
- What the medication is supposed to do (i.e., its action in understandable terms)
- Usual dosage and route of administration
- Potential serious adverse effects
- Common side effects
- Drug interactions
- Special nursing implications (e.g., whether it needs to be given with food or an hour after meals, whether sunlight should be avoided)

To reduce your fear of making a medication error, review the "Safety Guidelines to Prevent Medication Errors" in Chapter 5. If you understand how a drug works, you will be able to determine the possible side effects and nursing implications. When you are well prepared for each clinical experience, you will be less anxious, able to function in the clinical setting more efficiently, have less fear of hurting a patient, and learn more.

MOBILE DEVICES AND SOFTWARE

Some schools of nursing are recommending a portable handheld device (PHD) such as a smartphone, pocket PC (PPC), or tablet for use in the clinical setting. Depending on the model, these small computerized devices can store reference software, provide connection to the Internet, and have many apps and other add-on features. Software programs that are very helpful in clinicals include the following:

- Nursing diagnosis manual
- Guide to clinical procedures
- English-Spanish medical word and phrase program
- Guide to evidence-based practices
- Manual of diseases and disorders with specific information on assessments, nursing diagnoses, and management of commonly seen disorders
- Handbook of laboratory and diagnostic tests with nursing implications
- Drug guide
- Medical dictionary
- Links to published articles
- Calculator
- Databases
- Anatomy flash cards
- A textbook of medicine

■ NURSING CARE PLANS

After orientation you probably will be required to bring a written nursing care plan or concept care map for each clinical day. Some schools require a certain number of problem statements or nursing diagnoses to be worked out; others want a complete care plan for each patient. From the data gathering you did for your assignment, you will have the patient's medical diagnoses, diagnostic test data, some history, and nursing diagnoses or problems that were listed in the chart. Analyze your data and determine your own nursing diagnoses as you were taught in your fundamentals of nursing course.

Practical nursing (licensed practical nurse/licensed vocational nurse [LPN/ LVN]) students may be given the patient's problem statements/nursing diagnoses and asked to construct a plan from that point. Each problem statement/nursing diagnosis must be correlated with supporting data. Determine appropriate goals or outcome criteria for each diagnosis. Ask yourself whether the expected outcome you have written is measurable; in other words, will you be able to tell from evaluation data whether it has been met? When writing nursing care plans or designing concept care maps, you must pull together information you have learned from anatomy and physiology, microbiology, and psychology courses as well as your nursing courses, and must apply this information to a particular situation. Your fundamentals of nursing text plus the text for the specific clinical area to which you are assigned (e.g., obstetrics, medical-surgical, pediatrics, psychiatric) will provide information for usual problems and nursing actions for patients with the medical diagnosis or problems your patients have.

Nursing Diagnoses

Your school may not use nursing diagnoses as many health facilities do not use them. Other schools may still use them. Many nursing care plan books generalize nursing diagnoses and actions for a particular disorder. Your school bookstore may stock several. Choose one that is easy to understand and that is as close as possible to the format your school uses. Be aware, though, that you still must individualize the care plans for your patients. Many of these books have the care plans on a CD or website that you can individualize for your patients. Read through the plan listed and ask yourself whether each item applies to your specific patient before including it in your own nursing care plan. Nursing care planning is a thinking process, not simply a copying process. The whole idea is to systematically devise a plan to meet a patient's basic needs. It is best to look at patients holistically, including their psychosocial and physical needs. One way to check yourself when writing care plans is to see whether you have covered all areas of basic need. Box 2-1 offers a checklist for choosing nursing diagnoses using the acronym RN'S HOPE to ensure that you have considered all areas. **Two problems that students often overlook are limitations in self-care and lack of knowledge about the disease or its treatment**.

Each instructor views nursing care plans a bit differently, even within a particular school of nursing. Get to know what your instructor wants and how things should be worded in general. Ask to see an example of a nursing care plan that the instructor thinks is very good.

Interventions

Read your textbooks for ideas about actions that are appropriate to meet the patient's needs for each problem. For example, if the problem is potential infection related to poor nutritional status, then, in addition to monitoring for signs of infection—such as increased temperature; increased white blood cell count; redness, pain, and swelling of the wound; and purulent drainage—you would include actions to improve nutritional status. Such actions would be to increase protein and vitamin C intake and encourage a well-balanced diet with sufficient fluids and calories to maintain a positive nutritional balance. Of course, using good hand hygiene and aseptic techniques for dressing changes and using Standard Precautions are included as well. Actions must be individualized for each patient; actions for the patient who has diabetes might be a little different from those for a patient who does not.

Evidence-based practice should be the major focus for choosing interventions for your care plan or care map (see Chapter 6 for a list of suggested websites for searching the evidence).

Rationales

Many programs require a scientific rationale or principle for each action listed on your care plan. What is desired is a *science-based* reason to explain how the action works. An example for interventions included in the sample nursing care plan in Figure 2-1 is the following:

Intervention: Discourage intake of foods high in caffeine.
Rationale: The chemical caffeine causes blood vessels to constrict, increasing blood pressure.

Choosing Problem Statements/Nursing Diagnoses   BOX 2-1

Once you have analyzed your assessment data and selected the most obvious problems for your patient's nursing care plan, you should review each area of possible need to ensure that you have not missed an important area. One way to conduct this review is to keep in mind the acronym RN'S HOPE, which covers all areas of basic needs:

R Rest and activity
N Nutrition
S Safety
H Hygiene
O Oxygenation
P Psychosocial
E Elimination and education

Examples of nursing diagnoses grouped for problems for each area of basic need include the following:

REST AND ACTIVITY
- Activity intolerance
- Impaired physical mobility
- Fatigue
- Sleep deprivation
- Pain: acute or chronic

NUTRITION
- Risk for impaired liver function
- Imbalanced nutrition: less than body requirements
- Self-care deficit: feeding
- Risk for constipation
- Risk for unstable blood glucose level
- Impaired swallowing
- Fluid volume, deficient or excess
- Nausea
- Risk for electrolyte imbalance

SAFETY
- Acute confusion
- Contamination
- Risk for contamination
- Readiness for enhanced comfort
- Risk for injury
- Impaired physical mobility
- Risk for infection
- Impaired skin integrity
- Risk for impaired skin integrity
- Risk for peripheral neurovascular dysfunction
- Impaired verbal communication
- Hyperthermia
- Hypothermia
- Risk for falls
- Impaired memory
- Wandering

Continued

Choosing Nursing Diagnoses (cont'd)

HYGIENE

- Readiness for enhanced self-care
- Self-care deficit: toileting
- Self-care deficit: dressing
- Self-care deficit: bathing
- Impaired oral mucous membrane

OXYGENATION

- Ineffective airway clearance
- Risk for aspiration
- Risk for decreased cardiac tissue perfusion
- Ineffective breathing pattern
- Impaired gas exchange
- Ineffective peripheral tissue perfusion
- Decreased cardiac output

PSYCHOSOCIAL

- Ineffective coping
- Readiness for enhanced decision making
- Risk for compromised human dignity
- Interrupted family processes
- Fear
- Anxiety
- Disturbed body image
- Ineffective health maintenance
- Impaired home maintenance
- Readiness for enhanced hope
- Moral distress
- Readiness for enhanced power
- Chronic low self-esteem
- Spiritual distress
- Social isolation
- Stress overload

ELIMINATION AND EDUCATION

- Constipation
- Urinary retention
- Urinary incontinence, urge
- Urinary incontinence, stress
- Diarrhea
- Bowel incontinence
- Self-care deficit: toileting
- Fluid volume excess
- Sexual dysfunction
- Deficient knowledge

Some schools may use problem statements instead of nursing diagnoses. Remember that many nursing actions are used to prevent problems, and in this event these actions are grouped under a "risk for" nursing diagnosis. The three areas students most often overlook are self-care deficit, deficient knowledge, and the major reason the patient is in the hospital, such as fractured hip (impaired physical mobility) or myocardial infarction (decreased cardiac output). In addition, **each medication to be administered and each procedure to be performed should fit under some nursing diagnosis on the care plan as an intervention**.

NANDA International, Inc. Nursing Diagnoses: Definitions & Classifications 2015-2017, Tenth Edition. Edited by T. Heather Herdman and Shigemi Kamitsuru.
2014 NANDA International, Inc. Published 2014 by John Wiley & Sons, Ltd. Companion website: www.wiley.com/go/nursingdiagnoses.

Sample Nursing Care Plan

Selected nursing diagnoses, goals/expected outcomes, nursing interventions, and evaluations for a patient with hypertension

Situation: 53-year-old male with a blood pressure of 170/100 found during routine screening of all employees at a local plant. A visit to the hypertension clinic reveals that he is hypertensive, is 75 pounds overweight, smokes two packs of cigarettes a day, and eats snacks during the day and in the evening while watching television. The physician prescribes a low-sodium diet and a mild antihypertensive. During her interview with the patient, the nurse notes that he does not understand the nature of his illness, how his lifestyle is related to hypertension, and the purpose of the low-sodium diet and the expected action of the diuretic.

Nursing Diagnosis	Goals/Expected Outcomes	Nursing Interventions	Evaluation
Ineffective tissue perfusion related to increased peripheral vascular resistance *as evidenced by* BP, 172/102; P, 96; feet cool and pale; pedal pulses, 1+; capillary refill > 4s.	Patient will maintain adequate tissue perfusion as evidenced by: 1. BP within normal limits at end of 3 weeks. 2. Pulse returns to normal range within 4 weeks. 3. Skin of feet warm and dry within 4 weeks. 4. Capillary refill time less than 3 sec within 4 weeks. Patient will quit smoking within 1 month.	Teach to take antihypertensive as ordered; and monitor BP bid. Assess skin and peripheral pulses each visit. Discourage smoking; encourage him to quit smoking. Discourage intake of foods high in caffeine. Maintain sodium restrictions. Have patient weigh himself daily and keep record.	BP, 156/96; P, 86; skin on feet pale and cool; smoked only five cigarettes today; weight down 2 lbs. Continue plan.
Imbalanced nutrition, more than body requirements related to overeating and lack of exercise *as evidenced by* weight, 285 lbs; height, 6 ft; consumes lots of junk food between meals; no daily exercise program; watches a lot of television.	Patient will lose 2 lbs within 2 months. Consultation with dietitian within 2 weeks. Patient will maintain 2-lb/wk weight loss until normal weight of 210 lbs is attained. Patient will have developed daily exercise plan within 2 weeks.	Explain need to lose excess weight; encourage him to participate in weight loss plan. Assist with development of daily exercise plan. Ask for dietary consult.	Weight, 283 lbs; is considering options for daily exercise plan.

FIGURE 2-1 Sample nursing care plan.

Continued

Sample Nursing Care Plan—cont'd

Nursing Diagnosis	Goals/Expected Outcomes	Nursing Interventions	Evaluation
Deficient knowledge related to self-care aspects of hypertension: how to take blood pressure, medication rationale and side effects, low-sodium diet, need for exercise, need for continued medical follow-up *as evidenced by* lack of ability to take own blood pressure; unsure about new antihypertensive medications; unfamiliar with low-sodium diet; unaware of need for regular exercise to control weight and blood pressure; complaints of cost of going to the doctor.	Patient will demonstrate correct technique for taking own blood pressure within 1 week of teaching. Patient will explain action of antihypertensive medication and possible side effects 1 week after teaching session. Patient will describe effects of exercise on cardiovascular system after teaching session. Patient will state which foods are high in sodium when given a list from which to choose foods after teaching session. Before discharge patient will give three reasons why continued follow-up is necessary for patients with hypertension.	Develop teaching plan covering the following points: 1. How to take own blood pressure. 2. Action and side effects of antihypertensive medication. 3. Beneficial effects of exercise program on cardiovascular system. 4. How sodium increases water retention and elevates blood pressure. 5. Foods to avoid that contain excess sodium. 6. Potential complications of uncontrolled blood pressure and reasons for physician examination to detect beginning complications.	First teaching session completed; verbalizes action and three side effects of antihypertensive medication; can pick foods high in sodium from a list. Continue teaching and plan. Progressing toward outcomes.
Risk for ineffective coping related to lack of desire to quit smoking, even though he is hypertensive. *as evidenced by* lack of desire to quit smoking and that he doesn't really need to do so because all of his friends smoke.	Patient will verbalize how smoking affects the blood vessels 3 days after teaching session. Patient will verbalize desire to quit smoking within 1 month. Patient will institute a "no smoking" program within 1 month.	Teach how nicotine constricts the blood vessels, elevating blood pressure and decreasing blood flow to the periphery of the body. Encourage patient to quit smoking. Obtain both American Heart Association, American Lung Association, and American Cancer Society materials regarding the dangers of smoking. Familiarize the patient with available community "Quit Smoking" programs. Encourage him to join support group for those who are quitting smoking.	Discussed effect of smoking on vessels; gave patient AHA materials to read; encouraged him to quit smoking; scheduled another session tomorrow. Continue plan.

FIGURE 2-1, cont'd

A sample concept map or care map, sometimes used in place of a full nursing care plan, is illustrated in Figure 2-2.

EVALUATION

The evaluation section of the nursing process cannot be completed until you carry out your plan of care during clinical hours. After you have cared for the patient, go back and revise your preliminary plan. Some of the problem statements/nursing diagnoses you listed may not be pertinent, and you may have discovered other problems and concerns that are more important to the patient. Delete actions that are ineffective, and devise new ones to help meet your stated expected outcomes. Usually the care plan does not have to be recopied; you just add to it, perhaps in a different color ink to show what has been changed and updated.

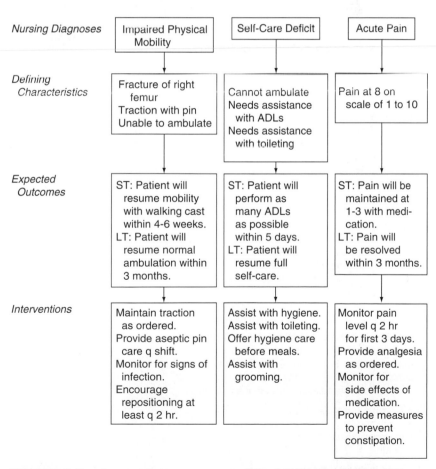

The Patient with a Fractured Femur

Nursing Diagnoses	Impaired Physical Mobility	Self-Care Deficit	Acute Pain
Defining Characteristics	Fracture of right femur Traction with pin Unable to ambulate	Cannot ambulate Needs assistance with ADLs Needs assistance with toileting	Pain at 8 on scale of 1 to 10
Expected Outcomes	ST: Patient will resume mobility with walking cast within 4-6 weeks. LT: Patient will resume normal ambulation within 3 months.	ST: Patient will perform as many ADLs as possible within 5 days. LT: Patient will resume full self-care.	ST: Pain will be maintained at 1-3 with medication. LT: Pain will be resolved within 3 months.
Interventions	Maintain traction as ordered. Provide aseptic pin care q shift. Monitor for signs of infection. Encourage repositioning at least q 2 hr.	Assist with hygiene. Assist with toileting. Offer hygiene care before meals. Assist with grooming.	Monitor pain level q 2 hr for first 3 days. Provide analgesia as ordered. Monitor for side effects of medication. Provide measures to prevent constipation.

FIGURE 2-2 Sample concept map or care map. *ADLs,* Activities of daily living; *LT,* long term; *ST,* short term.

PATHOPHYSIOLOGY STATEMENT

Some programs also require a pathophysiology statement concerning the patient's medical diagnosis or problem. For beginning courses, a simple explanation of the diagnosis, including the physiological changes the disease or disorder is causing and the signs and symptoms expected, is usually all that is necessary. **If the patient is undergoing or has undergone surgery, complete the pathophysiology statement on the disorder that necessitated the surgery**. Include the type of surgical procedure performed and the physiological changes that the patient has experienced.

In more advanced courses you should consider the course of the disease or disorder and the prognosis if there is no intervention. Determine what the potential complications of the disorder may be, and discuss the effect of the problem on the patient's basic needs. Box 2-2 provides two examples of pathophysiology statements. Figure 2-3 illustrates a pathophysiology concept map.

Writing pathophysiology statements helps you understand what is going on physiologically in the patient and how the condition is causing interference with

---

Examples of Pathophysiology Statements

BOX **2-2**

A pathophysiology statement usually consists of the etiology of the disease or disorder, the usual signs and symptoms in comparison with the individual patient's signs and symptoms, the usual treatment, and potential complications.

EXAMPLE 1: CHOLELITHIASIS

Cholelithiasis is the presence of gallstones in the biliary system. The stones may be located in the gallbladder, the common duct, or the hepatic ducts of the liver. The stones may consist of cholesterol, pigments (mainly unconjugated bilirubin), or a combination of these substances with calcium carbonate, phosphate, or bile salts. Gallstones occur more frequently in women, and the incidence increases with age. This patient has the following risk factors: obesity, diabetes mellitus.

Usual signs and symptoms include pain, often in the upper right quadrant; jaundice; nausea and vomiting; bloating and indigestion; and fatty food intolerance. This patient has upper midline pain radiating to the right shoulder blade, nausea, and an intolerance to fatty foods.

Treatment consists of surgically removing the stones or breaking up the stones with lithotripsy or by chemical dissolution. This patient underwent laparoscopic cholecystectomy.

Complications include residual stones in a duct causing blockage, infection from the surgical procedure, and internal bleeding from surgery.

EXAMPLE 2: MYOCARDIAL INFARCTION

Atherosclerosis → coronary thrombosis (or embolus) → occlusion of artery → myocardial tissue perfusion → impaired muscle function → (there should be an arrow indicating decreased here) → cardiac output*

Potential complications include the following:

- Necrosis of tissue
- Dysrhythmia
- Congestive heart failure
- Death

*Can be illustrated in the form of a concept map.

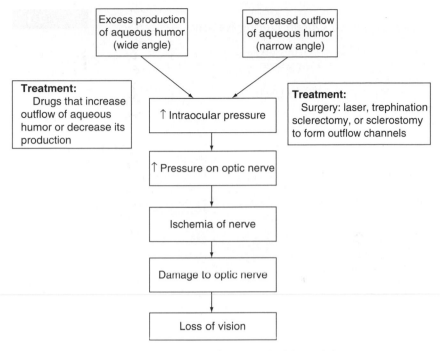

FIGURE 2-3 Concept map of the pathophysiology of glaucoma.

the patient's ability to provide for his or her own basic needs. That is where you put your nursing actions to work—you assist the patient in meeting basic needs when he or she is unable to do so. You can attempt to prevent complications that would extend the illness or delay the surgical recovery.

Together, your chart review, preparatory reading, pathophysiology statement, and construction of the preliminary nursing care plan provide you with most of the data you need to care adequately for your patient. You will add information from a shift report to help determine what care your patient will need that day.

Listening to the Shift Report

When listening to the morning or evening report (Box 2-3), you should write down pertinent information about your patients and all nursing care to be performed on your work organization sheet (Figure 2-4). If you did not understand something, ask the nurse in charge about it. Verify with the staff nurse who is assigned to your patient your understanding of what you are responsible for in the care of the patient, and **state those tasks that are beyond your skill level**. Make certain that the staff nurse understands that you do not perform tasks or assessments beyond your skill level. **This clarification is your responsibility**. Nurses work with students from different schools and different course levels. Unless you state differently, the nurse may assume you are doing everything that needs to be done for the patient, and vital assessments and treatments may go undone.

Information to Obtain During Report

BOX 2-3

- Room number and bed designation
- Date of admission and physician
- Diagnoses
- Current surgery or delivery and type:
  Vaginal or C-section
  Gravida
  Para
- Surgery or tests scheduled for next 24 hours
- Vital signs schedule
- Neurological signs schedule
- Abnormalities to report to physician
- Diet:
  NPO
  I&O previous shift
- Finger-stick glucose:
  • Insulin orders
- Tubes:
  • NG
  • Foley
  • Drains
- Oxygen:
  • Saturation
  • Cannula
  • Mask
  • Flow rate
  • PRN
  • Continuous
- IV location, type, when inserted:
  • Solution hanging
  • Amount left to count
  • Solution to follow
- Equipment:
  • Fetal monitor
  • SCD
  • CPM
  • Traction/type
  • PCA
  • Oximeter
  • Telemetry
  • Other

- Treatments:
  • Heat lamp
  • Sitz
  • Dressing changes
  • ROM
  • TCDB
  • Spirometer
  • Heat/cold
  • K-pad
- Type of bath:
  • Shower
  • Assist
  • Complete bed bath
- Activity:
  • OOB
  • BSC
  • BRP
  • BRP with assistance
  • Bed rest
- PRN medications given last shift
- Pain level:
  • Pain management
- Impairments:
  • Vision
  • Hearing
  • Paresis
  • Paralysis
  • Amputation (old/new)
- Mental status:
  • Alert
  • Confused
  • Comatose
- Medication changes
- Problems
- Concerns/need for order changes
- Needed teaching
- Psychosocial status
- Patient-family dynamics
- Amount of assistance needed

BRP, Bathroom privileges; *BSC,* bedside commode; *CPM,* continuous passive motion; *I&O,* intake and output; *IV,* intravenous; *NG,* nasogastric; *NPO,* nothing by mouth; *OOB,* out of bed; *PCA,* patient-controlled analgesia; *PRN,* as needed; *ROM,* range of motion; *SCD,* sequential compression device; *TCDB,* turn, cough, and deep breathe.

SHIFT WORK ORGANIZATION SHEET

PATIENT/ROOM	8:00	9:00	10:00	11:00	12:00	13:00	14:00	15:00
J.D. 521	V.S. Quick Assess	930 Shower 945 Adressing		Full Assess Chart	V.S. Glucometer	Pre-op teaching Chart	I + O Tape report	Close chart
R.S. 523¹	V.S. 820 Quick Assess √IV	Feed Full Assess √IV	Bathe + Bed √IV	Chart √IV	Feed √IV	Let Nap √IV	Empty Foley I + O √IV	Close chart √IV
B.W. 523²	V.S. Quick Assess √IV	Full Assess √IV	Shower + Bed √IV	Chart √IV	V.S. √IV	√IV	I + O √IV	Close chart √IV
PATIENT/ROOM								

FIGURE 2-4 Sample shift work organization sheet.

Continued

MEDICATION TIMES

PATIENT/ROOM	7:30	8:00	9:00	10:00	11:00	12:00	13:00	14:00	15:00	PRN
J.D. 521	Insulin	✓✓	✓✓ ✓✓			S.S. Insulin		✓		Pain 10^{40} 14^{10}
R.S. 523[1]			✓✓				✓✓			
B.W. 523[2]		✓	✓✓✓				✓			
PATIENT/ROOM										

FIGURE 2-4, cont'd

Preparing for Patient Teaching

From the patient assignment information and your reading about the disease process and nursing care, you will have an idea of the areas in which patient teaching may be required. If the patient will be having a diagnostic test, read about the test and especially note the pretest and post-test nursing care. If appropriate, ask to accompany the patient for the test to develop first-hand knowledge of what the patient experiences. This information will give you an edge in answering patient questions and help you know what to expect during your time of care. Having this information also helps with clinical time organization.

Other areas in which teaching may be necessary include self-care tasks such as cast care, dressing changes at home, diabetic self-care, medication administration, preoperative teaching, and any other health care–related task the patient and family will be performing at home. Teaching for home care should begin early in the patient's hospital stay. Useful materials for patient teaching can be found in your textbooks and on the Internet. Search by topic or visit one of the medical websites listed in Chapter 6. Useful diagrams or sets of instructions for self-care are sometimes available to give the patient.

Every patient must receive discharge teaching and instructions before being released from the hospital. Find out what the hospital requires and what materials are available in print or on the in-house TV system or Intranet. The topics covered are essentially the same for each patient, but the amount of instruction and the variations in care necessary at home depend on the patient's diagnosis or problem. Box 2-4 presents a checklist for discharge teaching so that you will be prepared if your patient is discharged on your clinical day.

Organizing Your Workday

Regardless of the number of patients you are taking care of, organize your workday. Decide what you are going to do at which times according to the priority of

---

BOX 2-4

Checklist for Discharge Teaching

Instructions must be given to each patient and family or significant other before discharge. Provide written instructions whenever possible in addition to verbal instructions, and cover the following topics:

Medications—Name, dosage, times to be taken, special instructions

Diet—What to eat, foods to avoid

Activity—Exercise, rest, lifting, stair climbing, driving, resumption of sexual activity; special instructions for use of crutches, cane, walker

Breathing exercises—Schedule for deep breathing and coughing or for incentive spirometry

Wound care—How to cleanse the wound and change the dressing, signs and symptoms to report

Bathing—Type of bath or shower permitted

Next contact with the physician—When to call for appointment or time of appointment

Signs and symptoms to report—Report temperature higher than 100.1° F, increase in pain, nausea and vomiting; particular instructions for individual patient

Special instructions—Any specific points necessary for proper self-care

the tasks. The shift report has given you data about the times that various things must be done. Vital signs are usually taken at 8:00 AM, 12:00 PM (noon), 4:00 PM, or 8:00 PM. If treatments are scheduled twice a day (bid) or three times a day (tid), you will have some flexibility in deciding when you wish them to be done (whether you can do them or not—consult your staff nurse). Consider whether the patient will be having physical therapy or special tests. Will the patient be off the unit or busy with the therapist? Ask the staff nurse. Plan what time you will bathe the patient, make the bed, and do your more complete physical assessment. When will you do the dressing change or have the patient ambulate? Plan the time for turning, deep breathing, supervised use of incentive spirometer, and coughing. Provide periods when the patient can rest. If you have several patients, plan your tasks in rotation so no one is neglected. Each patient should be seen at least every hour during the day shift. Initially, you will probably be assigned to only one patient. By the end of the first semester, you should be caring for at least two patients.

Figure 2-4 provides a sample shift work organization plan. A well-done shift work organization sheet provides a good guide by which to do your charting. At the end of each clinical day, review your work organization sheet to determine whether your plan worked. If it did not, think about what to change before you use the form again. Figure 2-5 is a sample of a patient care worksheet similar to that used by many nurses to jot down information during report.

Complying with HIPAA Requirements

Federal privacy regulations came into effect in April 2003 with the overall Health Insurance Portability and Accountability Act (HIPAA). The rules govern how patient information is conveyed, stored, and shared. Box 2-5 presents a synopsis of the major points. **You must not discuss anything about your patients or clients with anyone who is not directly involved in their care**. Refrain from talking about your patients with others assigned to the same unit in the elevators or the cafeteria, where you may be overheard. **If you are documenting via computer, do not leave the screen unattended while a patient record is viewable**. Refrain from writing patient names on your written work; use only initials. When performing patient teaching or answering questions, keep your voice low and provide as much privacy as possible. Do not allow anyone not directly involved in the patient's care to view the medical record. HIPAA gives patients the right to correct erroneous information in their records and the right to the information in the record. Follow the agency's procedure if the patient requests to see the medical record. In many instances the medical record is available to the patient only after discharge.

Cell phones are not to be used within the public areas of the hospital. It is not professional to carry on personal conversations during your clinical hours. Patients should never be discussed with others, including family, colleagues on other units, or with staff in the elevators. Never take pictures of anything on the patient unit with your cell phone camera. If you have a home emergency, ask permission to leave the floor and go to a private place to return the call. Otherwise wait until you are off duty and outside the premises or in a private area.

HIPAA law extends to any comments about a patient on the Internet. **You must not blog or comment about a patient in any way on social networking sites or your own blog, even if names are not used.** Do not discuss anything to do

PATIENT CARE WORKSHEET

PATIENT	ROOM #	DIAGNOSIS	V/S	DIET	I & O	ACTIVITY	MISC.

FIGURE 2-5 Patient care worksheet.

with a patient outside of the clinical unit or with anyone other than your clinical instructor.

Reviewing Basic Communication

Knowledge of the basic principles of therapeutic communication is essential for establishing rapport and trust and using specific techniques to facilitate interaction. Practice using therapeutic techniques whenever you can. Listen beyond the words, and look for the feelings the patient is trying to convey.

NONVERBAL CUES (WHAT TO WATCH FOR)

Watch for nonverbal communication in body posture, facial expression, gestures, hand movements, and foot swinging, among others. Ask yourself whether the nonverbal clues fit the words.

VERBAL CUES (WHAT TO LISTEN FOR)

Express interest in and encouragement for what the patient is saying. Nod your head, maintain eye contact, and say "uh-huh" or "mmm." Lean slightly toward the

---

BOX 2-5

Patient Rights and Provider Responsibilities Covered by the Health Insurance Portability and Accountability Act (HIPAA)

- Consent—Written consent must contain a clause that says the patient agrees to allow the provider to use and disclose his or her information for treatment, payment, and health care operations. A notice must be attached to the consent form.
- Notice—The provider's obligations are outlined regarding the privacy of the patient's health care information. It includes the six patient rights and the responsibilities of the provider. It details how the patient information will be protected and a process for filing a complaint if the patient believes privacy rights have been violated.
- Access—The patient has the right to inspect and copy his or her medical record.
- Amendment—A patient has the right to amend his or her record for the purpose of accuracy.
- Accounting for disclosures—Providers are held accountable for how a patient's medical information is handled. Tracking any disclosures of information that were not related to treatment, payment, or health care operations, or that were not authorized by the patient, must occur.
- Restriction of disclosure—The patient can request that the provider restrict the use and disclosure of his or her information. The provider does not, however, have to grant the request.

Adapted from deWit SC, O'Neill P: *Fundamental concepts and skills for nursing,* ed 4, Philadelphia, 2014, Saunders.

---

patient. Use reflection for the feeling you sense behind the words, and ask for feedback from the patient as to whether what you perceive is correct. For example, "I sense that you are unsure about what to do." Such a statement allows the patient to validate or correct your impression.

USING SILENCE
Use silence appropriately; it gives the patient time to gather thoughts and formulate a response. Summarizing the highlights and main ideas of the interaction gives the patient a chance to correct any misperceptions and to know clearly what has been relayed to the nurse.

ELICITING A RESPONSE
Use open-ended questions that will elicit more than a one- or two-word answer. Asking "who," "what," "where," or "how" requires the patient to elaborate when answering. Use "why" questions with caution and rarely; they tend to make the patient feel defensive. Table 2-2 provides examples of therapeutic communication techniques and barriers to communication.

HELPING THE PATIENT CHOOSE
Assist the patient to solve the problem. Do not give advice or opinions. Let the patient choose alternatives that appeal to him or her for solution of the problem.

TABLE 2-2 Quick Therapeutic Communication Review

Technique	Example	Rationale
Therapeutic Communication Techniques		
General leads	"Go on." "I see." "Uh-huh." "Please continue."	Encourage patient to continue or elaborate
Open-ended questions or statements	"Tell me more about that feeling." "I'd like to hear more about ..." "How did it start?"	Encourage patient to elaborate rather than answer in one or two words
Offering self	"I'm here to listen." "Can I help in some way?"	Shows caring, concern, and readiness to help
Restatement	*Patient:* "I tossed and turned last night." "You feel like you were awake all night?"	Restates in different words what the patient has said and encourages further communication on that topic
Reflection	*Patient:* "I'm so scared about the surgery; anesthesia terrifies me." "Can you tell me how anesthesia terrifies you?"	Reflecting same words back to patient. It also encourages further verbalization of feelings
Seeking clarification	*Patient:* "Seeing my little girl come visit me was so hard. I'm so upset." "Your daughter upset you?"	Seeks clarification if the little girl upset the patient or her leaving was the upsetting factor. Helps the patient clarify unclear thoughts or ideas
Focusing	"Do you have any questions about your chemotherapy?" "Let's look at your options."	Asking a goal-directed question helps the patient focus on key concerns
Encouraging elaboration	"Tell me what that felt like." "I need more information about that." "Tell me more about the experience."	Helps the patient describe more fully the concern or problem under discussion
Giving information	"The test results take at least 48 hours to return to us." "You will get a preoperative injection that will make you sleepy before you are taken into the operating room."	Informs the patient of information relevant to specific health care or situation
Looking at alternatives	"Have you thought about ...?" "You might want to think about ..." "Would this be an option?"	Helps patients see options and consider alternatives to make their own decisions about health care
Silence	*Patient:* "I don't know if I should have chemotherapy, radiation, or both." [Nurse remains silent]	Maintaining silence and sitting attentively but quietly allows patients time to gather their thoughts and sort them out

Continued

TABLE 2-2 Quick Therapeutic Communication Review (cont'd)

Technique	Example	Rationale
Summarizing	"You've identified your alternatives pretty clearly." "You are aware of the important signs and symptoms to report to your physician; plan to call to make an appointment next week."	Sums up the important points of an interaction

Blocks to Effective Communication

Technique	Example	Rationale
Changing the subject	*Patient:* "I'm so worried about my husband." "It is time for your bath now."	Deprives the patient of the chance to verbalize concerns
Giving false reassurance	"I'm sure it will turn out fine." "You don't need to worry."	Negates the patient's feelings and may give false hope, which, if things turn out differently, can destroy trust in the nurse
Judgmental response	"I don't think that was a good thing for you to do considering you have diabetes."	Implies that the patient must take on the nurse's values and is demeaning to the patient
Defensive response	*Patient:* "My doctor never seems to know what is going on." "Dr. Smith is a very good doctor; he's here every day."	Nurse responds by defending the doctor. Prevents patients from feeling that they are free to express their feelings
Asking probing questions	"Why were you there at that hour?" "What did you intend to prove?"	Pries into the patient's motives and therefore invades privacy
Using clichés	"Cheer up, you'll be home soon." "This won't hurt for long." "You have a long life ahead of you."	Negates the patient's individual situation; stereotypes the patient. This type of response sounds flippant and prevents the building of trust between patient and nurse
Giving advice	"If I were you, I would …" "I think you should …" "Why don't you …?"	Tends to be controlling and diminishes patients' responsibility for taking charge of their own health
Inattentive listening	Turning your back when the patient is sharing feelings or pertinent information; showing impatience with body language (i.e., tapping your foot or having your hand on the door to go out).	Indicates that the patient is not important, that the nurse is bored, or that what is being said does not matter

Adapted from deWit S, O'Neill P: *Fundamental concepts and skills for nursing*, ed 4, St Louis, 2014, Saunders.

Help explore what the alternatives might be, and then let the patient choose what is best.

Approaching the Patient

Plan your first approach to the patient. If you are entering to take vital signs, be certain that you have all your equipment with you, including a piece of paper on which to write the results. One way to approach the patient is, "Good morning, my name is _____, and I will be working with _____ (staff nurse) as your student nurse today." If it is the late shift, simply substitute "hello" for "good morning." Inquire how the patient slept last night or how the day has gone so far. Listen attentively. Express appropriate reactions or nod gently. Explain what you are going to do, and then do it.

To interview the patient and gather the data you need for your assessment, explain that you have looked at the chart but that your instructor requires that you ask a lot of questions that have probably already been asked by the physician or other nurses. Explain that a part of your learning experience is to interview the patient yourself. When you have gathered the data you need, perform a beginning quick assessment following the guidelines in Box 2-6. This type of quick assessment should be done within the first hour of your shift. You will be able to gather additional history and data about the patient as you interact with him or her throughout the shift. An in-depth physical assessment can be performed a little bit at a time during the shift.

Assisting with the bath provides a prime opportunity to develop rapport with the patient and to focus the conversation on his or her concerns. You can also conduct a significant amount of physical assessment at that time—skin condition, range of motion of joints, ability to follow instructions, and level of alertness and cognition, among others. Your priority is to keep the interaction focused on the patient and not on yourself. A fine balance exists between the social interaction the patient needs and the professional interaction you need.

Learning from the Staff

The unit secretary or clerk can be an ally if you are kind and friendly; you want this person "on your side." Address the person by name, and be considerate. Do not interrupt his or her work if you can help it.

The charge nurse is ultimately responsible for the patients on the unit. This is the person to consult about patient assignments and problems. However, it is the staff nurse you will work with most closely. This nurse may be a registered nurse (RN) or an LPN/LVN. In either case, this person can teach you a lot. Remember that nurses have different personalities, strengths, and weaknesses just like everyone else. Some staff nurses like working with students more than others. Which type of person you have on any given day is not predetermined. If the staff nurse likes to teach, use his or her expertise to the maximum. If you are finished with your patient care, ask whether you can shadow the staff nurse while he or she cares for other patients.

If you are working with a nurse who makes it obvious that a student is an inconvenience, simply stay out of the way, keep the nurse posted on assessments and tasks completed for your patient, and use your instructor as your primary resource for the day. The nurse may just be having a bad day or may have a patient who is not doing well, which may make him or her worried and preoccupied. It is not usually a personal reaction toward you. Talk with your instructor about your

BOX **2-6**

Quick Head-to-Toe Assessment

At the beginning of each shift, each patient should be assessed quickly. This assessment is often performed along with the vital signs.

INITIAL OBSERVATION
- Is the patient breathing?
- Skin color
- Appearance
- Affect
- How is the patient feeling?

HEAD
- Level of consciousness
- Appearance of eyes
- Ability to communicate
- Mentation status

VITAL SIGNS
- Temperature
- Pulse rate; rhythm
- Respiration rate, pattern, and depth
- Oxygen saturation
- Blood pressure (compare with previous readings)

PAIN LEVEL
- Use pain scale
- Determine location*

ABDOMEN
- Shape
- Soft or hard
- Bowel sounds
- Appetite
- Last bowel movement
- Voiding status

EXTREMITIES
- Normal movement
- Skin turgor and temperature
- Peripheral pulses
- Edema

TUBES AND EQUIPMENT PRESENT
- Intravenous catheter: condition of site, fluid in progress, rate, additives
- Oxygen cannula: liter flow rate
- Pulse oximeter: intact probe, readings
- Nasogastric tube: suction setting, amount and character of drainage
- Urinary catheter: character and quantity of drainage
- Dressings: location, drains in place, wound suction devices, character and amount of wound drainage
- Traction: correct weight, body alignment, weights hanging free
- External fixator, pin location appearance, drainage
- Other equipment (CPM, SCDs, etc.)

HEART AND LUNG ASSESSMENT
For patients with current or potential heart or lung problems, auscultation of the heart and lungs should be performed on the initial assessment. For patients without these problems, auscultation can be performed later in the shift.

CPM, Continuous passive motion; *SCD*, sequential compression device.
*Pain is assessed whenever vital signs are measured.

feelings. Try to remember the times when you have not wanted a younger sibling around or were angry with family members for one reason or another. Follow the correct lines of communication; however, do not skip giving this nurse information that is needed about the patient. Remember to "report off" to the nurse at the end of your shift.

When other health care professionals work with the patient, try to learn about what they are doing. Ask the respiratory therapist to show you more about the oxygen device in use. Watch the speech therapist work with the patient; then you can help the patient practice the exercises. Listen when the dietitian provides diet counseling, and you will be able to reinforce the teaching with the patient. Go with the physician when he or she visits the patient. Stay out of the way and observe. Ask any questions after you leave the room.

Staying in the Good Graces of Your Instructor

Find out exactly what your instructor expects of you in the clinical area, and question any instructions you do not understand. Most instructors expect the following:

- Thorough preparation for the clinical and lab experiences
- Written work that is legible and neat
- A professional, clean, crisp appearance and demeanor
- A friendly, quiet, professional demeanor
- Sufficient sleep before the clinical experience
- Promptness for clinical and conference
- Active participation in clinical conference
- A quick report on your patients when approached during the shift
- Cooperative, team attitude with the staff
- Attentiveness to patient needs
- Appropriate and complete documentation
- Attentive listening and attention to instructions
- Seeking of skill experiences
- Taking responsibility for your own learning
- To find you in the patients' rooms when you are not charting, rather than sitting at the nurses' station
- You ask questions when you do not know how to do something or whether it is permissible for you to do it
- To be notified immediately if something untoward happens or if a mistake is made

Recall that the role of the instructor is to correct and instruct you; do not take every comment made by the instructor as a personal attack. Some are better at gently correcting than others. Your instructor is there to prevent you from harming a patient. The instructor is your safety net. If you happen to have an instructor whom you cannot seem to please, make an appointment to talk about it. Ask what you can do to make the situation better. Tell him or her how you are feeling; your instructor is there to help you.

Preventing Errors and Harm to Patients

Always be attuned to patient safety factors. When the bed is raised, keep side rails up when you are not at the bedside. Remember to lower the bed when you have finished working with the patient and lower side rails per agency protocol. Always turn around when leaving the room and survey it. Does the patient have the call bell within reach? Are the items needed within reach?

Do not attempt to move an incapacitated patient by yourself unless you are certain you can manage the correct technique for a safe transfer. Get help—it is not worth the risk of hurting the patient or yourself. You, in turn, can help others on the unit to move their patients. Learn to use the patient lifts that are available.

If you are told that a tube or IV cannula is to be removed from your patient, always check the chart and **read the actual order before taking the tube out**. Re-inserting a tube or IV cannula that was withdrawn in error is not fun, and it subjects the patient to unnecessary discomfort and risk of infection.

Follow the accepted six *rights* (see Chapter 5), *five responsibilities*, and *three checks* method for administering medications. Perform the first two medication checks in the medication room or at the cart. Take the medication administration record (MAR) to the patient along with the medications, and check the identification armband immediately on approaching the patient. Use an additional identifier (e.g., date of birth). Then check each medication appropriately with the MAR a third time just before administering it to the patient. Document that the medication has been given only after the patient has taken it. Use bar coding on the patient's bracelet and on the single-dose drug container as an added safety measure when it is available.

Immediately **report** abnormalities in vital signs to the staff nurse assigned to the patient. Discuss anything else you find unusual or of concern about the patient. Talk with your instructor about your concerns as well. It is better to have a concern checked out than to assume it is probably nothing to worry about.

Always report to the nurse when you leave the unit for a meal so that someone else will check on your patients while you are gone. Be certain your charting is caught up before you leave the floor.

Reviewing Documentation

There are many different systems of documentation within clinical facilities today (Box 2-7). You should receive information about the particular system used in your clinical facility and some guidelines for charting. If you do not receive this information, ask for it. There should be a charting or documentation manual available on the unit or on the facility intranet. You may be documenting on the computer or using a documentation simulation system on your school's intranet such as SIMChart. Your documentation of patient care is a legal record; it must be comprehensible, objective, neat, and complete.

It is best to organize before beginning to enter your nurse's notes. Chart from an outline format or chart from the data on your work organization sheet. Much information is recorded on flow sheets in the chart or electronic record, such as the graphic record for vital signs, intake and output (I&O) sheet, daily activity or daily assessment form, IV flow sheet, and MAR. However, in any documentation system, any abnormal findings must be recorded in the nurse's notes along with a description of the action taken to correct the problem.

Most hospitals require that a nurse document data for each nursing diagnosis, problem, or "need" in the patient's chart or electronic record at least once every 24 hours. For the nursing student, assessment data and actions should be recorded

Types of Documentation for Nurse's Notes

BOX 2-7

SOURCE-ORIENTED OR NARRATIVE CHARTING

Phrases and sentences are written out without any standardized structure, content, or form. Care given is documented in chronologic order. Assessments usually follow a body systems format. Portions of lines are not left blank.

Example

4/10/12 0830 States has an increasing ache at a 6 on a scale of 1 to 10 in the right hip. Began after being in the chair for breakfast. T. 98.4, P 82, R 16, BP 138/88. Unrelieved by position change.
0845 Vicodin tab × 1 PO
0940 States pain has decreased to a 3.

R. Sims, RN

PROBLEM-ORIENTED MEDICAL RECORD CHARTING FOR PROGRESS NOTES

All health care personnel chart on the same forms and sequentially as care is given. A *SOAP* format is used (**S**—*subjective* information, **O**—*objective* data, **A**—*assessment* data/impression, **P**—*plan*). Some agencies modify to a *SOAPIE* or *SOAPIER* format that adds **I**—*implementation*, **E**—*evaluation*, and/or **R**—*revision*.

Example

4/12/12 1000 Pain, chronic
S "The pain in my lower back is getting worse. It is a 7 on a scale of 1 to 10. It increased after I walked in the hall."
O Forehead furrowed. Legs pulled up toward body. P 88, R 18.
A Increased lumbar back pain.
P Medicate with oxycodone as ordered.

T. Munoz, RN

PIE CHARTING

PIE charting is an offshoot of SOAP charting. After designating the problem in one column, the note is formatted as **P**—*problem* identification, **I**—*interventions*, and **E**—*evaluation*.

Example

4/13/12 1420
P States pain has increased with inspiration and it hurts to deep breathe or cough.
I Medicated with albuterol inhaler 2 puffs at 1430.
E Pain eased by 1445. Able to complete use of incentive spirometer and to cough.

J. Porter, RN

FOCUS CHARTING

Focus charting is directed at a nursing diagnosis, a patient problem, a concern, a sign, a symptom, or an event. There are three components to the note: **D**—*data*, **A**—*action*, **R**—*response*. (**E** may be used instead of **R** and stands for *evaluation*.)

Example

4/14/12 1300 Impaired skin integrity right heel
D Heel red with 2-cm abrasion at base.
A Cleansed with sterile saline and applied Tegaderm.
R 2200 redness subsiding.

T. Moran, RN

Continued

Types of Documentation for Nurse's Notes (cont'd)

CHARTING BY EXCEPTION
Charting by exception assumes that all standards of practice are carried out and met with a normal or expected response *unless otherwise documented.* Documentation is done on a set of flow sheets, and a longhand note is written only when the standardized statement on the form is not met.

ELECTRONIC CHARTING
Electronic charting is done by scrolling through a variety of flow sheets on the computer and indicating care given and essential data about the patient. All entries to the patient record are done on-screen. There are several software systems for electronic charting in use.

for each problem dealt with during the shift. General guidelines are listed in Box 2-8.

If the hospital or clinical site is using an electronic medical record (EMR) system and the facility allows computer documentation by students, you will need to plan time to go through the training for use of that system. When training is complete, you will receive a password to access the system. Carefully read over what you have entered before pressing the Enter key or "OK." Your log-on name and password constitute your electronic signature. Log off the computer properly. **Never leave a computer without logging off.** Never enter data when someone else is logged on, and do not let anyone else use the computer when you are logged on. Keep the computer screen out of the view of visitors to protect the patient's privacy.

Giving a Report

When you leave your assigned unit for the day, you must "report off" to each nurse in charge of the patients assigned to you. If a nurse is on break when you are about to leave, "report off" to the charge nurse and make certain it is understood that you have not given your report to the primary nurse for the patient. Box 2-9 provides an outline of the information you should supply to each primary nurse for your assigned patients.

■ DEVELOPING PROFESSIONALISM

Nursing as a profession is striving to establish and maintain a professional image in the eyes of the public. The image you project as a nursing student and then as a nurse contributes to the overall public image of nursing. For this reason, nursing instructors will be teaching you about professionalism; they also will be evaluating you on your professional behavior. Image has three basic components: (1) appearance, (2) behavior, and (3) verbalization.

Appearance

Appearance includes clothes and grooming. Beside wearing the required uniform components, their cleanliness and neatness contribute to your image. Underwear should not be visible beneath a uniform, slips should not show beneath the skirt hem, buttons should not be missing, pocket corners should not be torn loose, hose should not have runs, shoes should be polished, shoelaces should be clean, and

BOX 2-8

Documentation (Charting) Guidelines

Think of your charting as a camera that takes the patient's picture.

ORGANIZE YOUR THOUGHTS
- What have I seen that relates to this problem?
- What have I done about it?
- What do I plan to do about it?
- How has my patient responded to what has been done?
- Do I have the right chart?

BUILD YOUR PLANNING ON YOUR:
- Initial assessment and further findings
- Identification of the patient's problems
- Patient care

GENERAL GUIDELINES
1. Chart neatly, legibly, and in black ink.
2. Be brief, concise, accurate, and complete.
3. Use good grammar, correct spelling, correct punctuation, and proper terminology.
4. Note the time of each entry; in addition, include the month, day, and year at the beginning of the shift charting.
5. Use a new line for each "new" (timed) entry. Draw an ink line through the extra space on a line you are charting if you have not used the entire line.
6. DO NOT ERASE. Draw a single line through an error; write "incorrect," "error," or "mistaken entry" over it; and sign your initials and the date (check agency procedure). Where room is available in the margin or above the corrected error, note the reason for it (e.g., wrong chart).
7. When correcting or making a change to an entry in a computerized system, enter the current time and date, identify yourself, and note the reason for the change.
8. Never chart in advance of doing something; in particular, do not chart medications before they are administered.
9. Include your signature and student designation (e.g., SN). Use your first initial and last name with that designation.
10. Leave out the word *patient*. If the meaning of the entry is ambiguous, use the patient's name.
11. Use only those abbreviations accepted in your agency. (See the documentation guidelines for the agency.)
12. Retain recopied pages in the back of the chart (i.e., corrected graphic record).
13. Check on the correct format for charts in your clinical facility.
14. Use flow sheets whenever possible—do not duplicate the information in the nurse's notes.
15. Use easily defined terms (e.g., "ate 75% of meal," rather than "ate well").
16. Rather than "tolerated well," state outcome: tolerated without pain, without nausea, or without complaint. (*Well* means different things to different people.)
17. At the end of your shift, check through your charts to ensure that notes are complete, that entries on flow sheets are finished, and that each note is signed. Check through medication administration records (MARs) for your assigned patients, and make certain that no medication has been overlooked and that you have initialed every medication you administered.

Continued

Documentation (Charting) Guidelines (cont'd)

CONTENTS TO INCLUDE

Body care: type of bath, back care, skin care and assessment, mouth care, hair care, perineal care, position changes (most data go on flow sheets)

Intake: diet, amount eaten as a percentage, fluids (oral, nasogastric [NG], intravenous [IV]); IV site condition, type of fluid, equipment changed, complaints (use activity sheet, intake and output [I&O] sheet, IV flow sheet)

Output: emesis, bowel movement, wound drainage, tube drainage, urine, vaginal flow, perspiration; include amounts and appearance (I&O sheet, nurse's notes)

Treatments: time, type, duration, appearance of area treated, special equipment, specifics of procedures, how it is done, patient response; if left unit, time left and by which conveyance, time returned

Tests: laboratory specimens drawn; cultures, disposition of specimens, radiographs, sonograms, endoscopies, patient reaction, outcome if known; time left and returned to floor

Dressings: appearance of incision or wound, smell, presence of drainage and appearance, how redressed and by whom

Activity: time, ambulation and distance, exercises performed, including leg and breathing postoperatively, range of motion (ROM) performed, physical therapy, condition of pressure points, repositioning and for how long, and patient response to each

Oxygen: time applied or amount changed, method of administration, safety precautions

Medications: time, amount, route, response, any adverse reaction or side effects, omission or delay, evidence of expected action (as needed [PRN] and immediate [STAT] doses are charted on the MAR and in the nurse's notes)

Sleep: day or night; amount, interruptions; patient comments

Mental state (be objective): mood, level of consciousness, general behavior

Preoperative preparation: teaching, physical preparation, time and by whom; patient questions

Special conditions: traction; cast; special equipment, time applied, amount of weight, condition of patient, circulation checks and findings, skin condition, smell

Vital signs: temperature, pulse, respiration, blood pressure

Physician's visits: examinations, treatments

Visitors: who, how long, patient reaction

Feelings: what patient states regarding feelings, complaints, concerns

Physical assessment: what you see, hear, smell, and feel; auscultation of lungs, heart, bowel sounds, palpation of abdomen and pulses; inspection of skin; assessment of problem area in depth

Safety factors: side rails up or down, replaced after working with patient; warnings; security devices in place

shoes should have quiet soles. Depending on agency and school policy, visible tattoos and piercings may not be permitted.

Personal grooming of hair, beard, nails, and skin integrates with attire to project the visual image. The professionally groomed image includes keeping skin clean; wearing an effective, nonperfumed deodorant; and keeping nails clean and trimmed. Long nails make patients uneasy and are known to harbor bacteria. Infection control guidelines require that nail length be no more than one quarter inch. Nail extenders or false nails are not to be worn because they carry bacteria.

Giving a Report	BOX **2-9**

Organize your thoughts using an outline format before giving your report to the staff nurse assigned to your patient. Provide the following information briefly and professionally:

- Patient name and room number
- Condition of patient (any changes), last vital signs, oxygen saturation
- Diagnostic tests or surgery undergone or both
- Treatments or procedures performed (including bath)
- As-needed (PRN) medications given and effect
- Intake and output (I&O) if ordered
- Amount left to count in intravenous (IV) administration bag
- Appearance of IV sites and locations
- Tubes in place and whether functioning properly; output
- Appearance of wounds and dressings in place; wound drainage output
- Bowel sounds; present or absent?
- Whether patient has had a bowel movement
- Voiding status
- Any abnormalities of heart or lung sounds
- Pain or comfort status
- Any patient concerns
- *Use the SBAR format as appropriate: situation, background, assessment, recommendation*

For men, the face should be clean shaven or the beard neatly trimmed. For women, makeup should be minimal and low key, and nail polish should be clear or light in color and not be chipped. For both genders, hair should be secured so that it does not swing over the patient while you are performing care and should not have unnatural colors. Hair contains bacteria that can fall on the patient. Jewelry also harbors microorganisms; only a plain wedding band and watch should be worn in the clinical areas. Other types of rings and bracelets may injure the patient's skin while the nurse is giving direct care; further, you may lose a stone or break a bracelet if it catches on something. A good guideline is not to wear any jewelry that dangles or makes noise. Perfumed lotions or colognes should not be used, because they tend to cause nausea in people who are ill. Patients have a "clean and crisp" image of nurses, and they judge the nurse's competence by looks and behavior.

SMOKING
If a nursing student smokes during a break, a breath freshener should be used before returning to the bedside; the smell of cigarettes is offensive to an ill non-smoker. Cigarette smell is also carried on clothes back into patient areas. It is unprofessional to subject an ill person to this odor. Many facilities are completely smoke free and have no smoking areas. It might be a good time to quit the habit.

DRESS
Student nurses are expected to dress professionally whenever they enter the clinical facility. This includes if students need to go to the units to obtain the data needed for their patient assignments. Although uniforms are not usually required when

you are going to the hospital to gather patient data, a clean, pressed laboratory coat worn over professional clothes and a name tag are required. Jeans, shorts, miniskirts, T-shirts with slogans, sandals, spiked high-heeled shoes, cowboy boots, and other such casual attire are inappropriate.

It is not considered professional to wear a nursing uniform when out with friends for a drink or shopping after the day's work is done. People do not know whether you have just finished a shift or are about to go on duty. A uniform worn while working in a clinical setting can be contaminated with many types of bacteria. It is best to change before running errands on the way home. The uniform should be worn only to and from the clinical area or work and while you are on duty. A freshly laundered uniform is to be worn each clinical day.

Behavior

Behavior can add to your professional image or detract from it. Your facial expression, body language, and posture are components of your overall image. Chewing gum or eating while providing patient care is considered unprofessional. A cheerful smile, modulated voice, erect posture, and body language that indicate attentive listening and quiet efficiency instill a feeling of confidence in patients.

PREPARATION

Professional behavior also includes being well prepared for the clinical experience and turning in completed written work when it is due. Instructors expect students to come to the clinical experience on time, in correct attire, and with the tools of the trade—a working watch, a stethoscope, a pen, and a name tag and badge.

ENVIRONMENTAL NEATNESS

Attention to environmental care of the assigned patients' units and to the nurses' stations and workrooms is another facet of professional behavior. Patient areas should be straightened at least once a shift. When time permits, add water to flowers to keep them fresh. Clean up after yourself in the medication room and at the nurses' station. Wipe up spills, throw away trash, and put equipment back where it belongs.

ATTENDANCE AND PUNCTUALITY

Most nursing instructors consider the clinical experience equivalent to reporting to work. Absence is excused only for illness or a family emergency. It is not professional to miss your clinical day to study for an examination or to take care of outside business matters. However, students are expected to remain at home if they are ill with a condition that is contagious, such as a cold with fever, constant sneezing, coughing, or runny nose. Intestinal influenza symptoms of vomiting or diarrhea should also signal the student to stay home. Exposing patients or colleagues to additional illness is not professional. Know how to notify your instructor that you will not be in attendance.

COST CONTAINMENT

Think cost effectively. Return equipment no longer being used by patients quickly, and see to it that charges for its use are stopped. Do not use a plastic medicine cup if a paper one will serve the same purpose. Check the patient's room for needed dressing or procedure supplies before taking new items from the clean supply area, to ensure that the least amount of supplies is used. Continually ask yourself whether there is a less expensive way to do the procedure. Remember to charge out supplies you use for the patient as required.

Verbalization

Appropriate verbalization is the third component of the professional image. Stress is usually high for the nursing student when in the clinical setting. It is necessary to make a conscious effort to stop and think before speaking when under such stress. Try to develop some quick stress relief techniques that you can use to calm yourself in particularly stressful situations (see Chapter 3). When you are with patients or staff, it is better to say too little than too much. Be aware of any nervous habits you might have, such as talking too much or too loud, or giggling, and curtail the behavior when it starts.

PATIENT PRIVACY

Remembering to provide privacy when interviewing a patient or performing a procedure builds trust between the patient and the nurse. Keeping your voice low when in the halls or at the nurses' station helps maintain the restful atmosphere that patients need. Try to provide maximum privacy in semi-private rooms when interviewing a patient.

COURTESY

Be courteous to other health care workers, as well as to patients. Saying, "May I," "Please," and "Thank you," and refraining from directly interrupting another contribute to a professional image. Call the patient Mr., Mrs., or Ms. unless given permission to use his or her first name. Do not use "honey," "dear," or other such terms. Consideration of others is essential to professional behavior. You are there to meet the patient's needs, not to socialize. Keeping conversation and attention focused on the patient rather than on you or outside activities is best. Students should not gather together during clinical hours. Time is to be spent with the patients, studying their charts, or interacting with other health care professionals for the purpose of collaboration or learning.

NONJUDGMENTAL ATTITUDE

Another aspect of professionalism is development of a nonjudgmental attitude toward patients and staff. Students sometimes find fault with nurses who do things differently from how their nursing school is teaching them. There are many right ways to perform different tasks. If the principles of asepsis and safety are followed, there is nothing wrong with performing a procedure in a different sequence or in a different way. Before loudly proclaiming that a nurse is doing something wrong, it is wise to discuss the matter quietly with the instructor.

CULTURAL SENSITIVITY

Patients and staff are not to be judged according to the student's values or cultural beliefs. Through the clinical learning process, students will become familiar with and learn to respect the values and beliefs of other cultures and individuals. To care for patients of different cultures, you must learn about the practices of cultural groups other than your own. By inquiring about cultural practices you observe, you can learn a great deal. There are many articles on usual practices within a variety of cultural groups. Several practical handbooks are also available. Assessment of cultural preferences should be part of your nursing care. Never assume that just because a patient is part of an ethnic group he or she adheres to that group's cultural practices. You must assess rather than assume.

REPORTING PROBLEMS

If something has occurred with a patient that violates the principles of asepsis or safety, pointing it out to the instructor is the professional response. Current peer review criteria require that questionable practices or incidents be brought to the attention of the nurse involved and the supervisor. However, when you are in the student role, allowing the instructor to handle such matters is best.

HONESTY

Honesty is essential to professionalism. Students are encouraged to admit mistakes and be honest with everything that they do, including their written work. It is unprofessional to compose someone else's nursing care plans or other written assignments or to have others contribute to yours. There are times when good students are encouraged to assist those having trouble with written work. Discuss the guidelines for this type of activity with the instructor before giving or getting assistance.

Professional behavior includes resisting passing along information on test questions to students in other class sections or allowing other students to copy from your answers. Such behavior is considered as much a form of cheating as copying answers from another student's examination.

Incorporating professionalism into your behavior and nursing practice occurs over time. You will benefit from observing the image, behavior, and verbalization of nurses whom you perceive as being highly professional and then attempting to model yourself accordingly.

■ CLINICAL EVALUATION

Each nursing school has a form used to evaluate student performance in the clinical setting. Become familiar with this form during the first week of the semester. In addition, find the list of clinical objectives for the semester and review them each week to be sure you are meeting them.

Basic Competence

Initially, students are evaluated on their mastery of basic competence for particular skills. There often is a formal check-off evaluation period for various required skills in the skills laboratory before the student ever attempts the skill in the clinical setting. Usually a skill is either passed or failed. If the student does not pass the skill check-off evaluation, remediation and practice are necessary before a second chance is given to pass the skill.

Once the student is caring for patients in a clinical setting, informal evaluation takes place on a weekly basis. This means that students are evaluated for competence and consistency of correct performance of skills previously evaluated in the skills laboratory or for adherence to principles taught in the lecture class. (Some schools do not have a skills laboratory.) General concepts that are always undergoing constant evaluation, once they have been covered in theory class, include the use of medical asepsis, communication, safety, legalities of practice, organization, and time management.

As content regarding various body systems is covered in theory class, the instructor will be evaluating your ability to apply the principles you have learned in the clinical setting. For example, once you have covered the basic concepts of disease and nursing care for the urinary system, you will be expected to be able to assist a patient to urinate, check for a full bladder, realize when a patient has gone too long without emptying the bladder, recognize signs that might indicate an infection, and determine when the color of urine is abnormal. **Students sometimes fail to understand that they are going to be evaluated on synthesis and application of knowledge as well as on the performance of skills.**

If you have difficulty in the clinical area and very often find that things do not seem to be going right, immediately ask your instructor to meet with you to find out specifically what you can do to redirect the course of events. Admitting mistakes, taking positive steps to correct deficiencies, and being honest will cause your instructor to evaluate you on your progress rather than on individual situations during which things went wrong. In other words, you will be seen in a favorable light when you exhibit these behaviors.

Instructors often verbally tell students how they are doing every few weeks; if you do not get this type of feedback, ask for it. Try asking, "How am I doing? Is there any area in which you see that I need to improve to be at a passing level?" This feedback will help you relax more and stop worrying about what the instructor may be thinking.

Clinical Written Work

The evaluation of clinical written work is based on instructor expectations and course requirements. Items on the evaluation form usually indicate what will be evaluated on written work. For example, "Writes individualized problem statements/nursing diagnoses pertinent to each patient's condition and problems" may be one item on the evaluation form. This requirement is appropriate for a first-semester student. Progress toward meeting this requirement is shown by writing one or two correct problem statements or nursing diagnoses on the first nursing care plan, writing two or three correct problems on the next care plan, and writing correct problem statements/nursing diagnoses covering all of the patient's basic needs for the final care plan of the semester.

By the final course, the evaluation form might state, "Writes comprehensive problem statements/nursing diagnoses in order of priority for assigned patients, considering psychosocial aspects of care as well as physical condition and problems."

It is helpful to ask your instructor for a sample of the type and level of written work desired. This sample provides you with an image of what is expected. Each nursing instructor has particular ideas about how the various parts of the nursing care plan should be written. Some instructors place more emphasis on one part than on another. It is to your benefit to find out specifically what each instructor wants before you turn in your first assignment.

If there is a grading form to be used for the written work you are going to turn in, consult it to see that you have included everything that is required before completing the assignment. You do not want to lose points simply because you forgot to complete a section of the assignment.

Formal Evaluation

A formal, summary type of evaluation is usually performed at midterm and at the semester's end. At these times, the instructor will fill out the evaluation form and set a conference time to review it with you. Often you will be asked to perform a similar self-evaluation. Asking at the beginning of the semester whether a learning period and a specific evaluation period will be offered is best; you will then know what to expect. At formal evaluation time, you will be evaluated on your achievement of the objectives for the clinical experience as well as for each item on the evaluation form. Usually a minimum level of competency is expected from students at each level. This level is often defined by the course objectives. Instructors look for progress toward the course objectives as well as for consistency in adherence to the principles taught. If you do not feel that you understand the evaluation form, ask for a conference with your instructor during the first 2 weeks of school to clarify what is required of you.

DEALING WITH STRESS

3

■ CONTROLLING STRESS LEVELS

Becoming a nursing student automatically increases stress levels because of the complexity of the information to be learned and applied and because of new constraints on time. There are several ways you can consciously decrease the stress associated with school. One way is to become very organized so that assignment deadlines or tests do not come as sudden surprises. By following a consistent plan for studying and completing assignments, you can stay on top of requirements and thereby prevent added stress. Carry as few units as possible to lighten the study load.

Set Priorities

Another way to decrease stress while in school is to set personal priorities. Take time to survey all outside obligations and determine what can be given up during nursing school. Perhaps it would be best to concentrate solely on school if you are single and, if married or a parent, on school and family. That may mean restricting your social life or giving up many social activities such as being a scout leader, Sunday school teacher, room mother at school, chief carpool driver, soccer coach, or Little League organizer. When school is completed, these extra roles can be taken up again. Adopt the motto "Keep It Simple" for your life while in school. The fewer outside distractions and responsibilities you have, the better your chances for success. Do not let housemates or dorm mates constantly distract you.

Ask for Help

If you have home responsibilities, consider asking for assistance from family and friends during your school years. A lot of stress can be reduced if someone else will take over carpool duties for school-age children. Relatives and good friends may be willing to help with this task. A spouse may be able to help if work schedules permit. Relatives can act as representatives once in a while at a child's school function that falls on the evening before an important test. All household members can help with housekeeping, cooking, and errands. Adolescents can grocery shop from a list, and children from the age of 9 years can prepare a simple dinner, even if it is hot dogs, scrambled eggs and biscuits, or frozen dinners cooked in the microwave oven. Children can prepare their own school lunches and can fix yours, too! Things do not have to be perfect for these few years of school. Let go of ideals regarding meals and the state of living quarters or yard. The goal is to keep all occupants healthy and in touch with one another while you get through school. When a relative or dear friend asks what you would like for a special occasion gift, tell them you would like a maid service to clean the house really well or a gardener to do some yard work or to take care of some other major chore. Be creative with gift requests; ask for what you really need to decrease your stress.

Tackle One Task at a Time

Try to decrease your workload and maximize your time by handling items only once. Most of us spend a lot of time picking up things we put down rather than putting them away when we have them in hand. Going straight to the closet with your coat when you come in instead of throwing it on a chair saves you the time of hanging it up later. Discarding junk mail immediately and filing the rest of your bills and mail as they come in rather than creating an ever-growing stack saves time when you need to find something quickly. Filing all items requiring further attention in some fashion helps you remember to take care of things on time rather than being so engrossed in your schoolwork that you forget about them. Many nursing students have had their power or telephone service cut off because the bill simply was forgotten or buried in a pile of old mail.

Exercise

Regular exercise, even if only a 10-minute brisk walk each day, aids in reducing stress. Although you may have been able to enjoy regular sessions at the health club or at an exercise class several times a week, you now may have to cut down on that time without giving up a set schedule for an exercise routine. Using an exercise bicycle that has a book rack on it at home, the YMCA, or a health club can help you accomplish two goals at once. You can exercise while beginning a reading assignment or while studying notes for an exam. Listening to lecture recordings while doing floor exercises is another option. At least a couple of times a week, however, the exercise routine should be done without the mental connection to school; time for the mind to unwind is necessary, too.

Stop for 10 Minutes

Taking 10 minutes a day for yourself is very beneficial for stress reduction. Closing yourself in your room, lying down with eyes shut, and just free floating for a few minutes can revive energy and stop the whirlwind of thoughts of family obligations or nonstop tasks that tend to increase stress. Reading a few pages of a magazine or a book, listening to favorite music, napping for a short time, or doing a relaxation technique between the time you reach home and begin the evening routine can refresh both the body and the mind.

Focus on Now

Another technique to help keep stress levels at a minimum is to stop worrying about things that cannot be changed. A great deal of energy is spent by many people on worrying about a situation that has not yet taken place. There will be time enough to worry about an event once it has actually occurred. Check yourself and ask whether you are a person who spends precious energy in this fashion. Wouldn't you rather spend that energy elsewhere? All of your "preworry" most likely will not change the event. Worrying about whether your teenager will have an accident while driving will not prevent such an event or cause it to happen. Worrying about whether a completed assignment will be graded favorably will not affect the grade; what is done is done. Try to focus on this day and this time, and do not worry about problems ahead of time. Deal with problems as they occur; if you cross a bridge before you need to, you will be paying the toll twice.

Change Your Perception

Donald Tubesing, in his book *Kicking Your Stress Habits* (1992), talks about using the technique of relabeling (reframing) to alter stress from bad to good. (This book is still in print.) The author explains that the effect of an experience on you is determined by how you label it. You have a choice as to how you view things. Labeling your clinical experience as exciting and challenging will make it far less stressful than labeling it as frightening and forbidding. If you label events as adverse during your daily crises, you end up with a batch of problems by the end of the day; if you label the same events as challenges, you end up with a bunch of opportunities. When something really seems stressful, ask yourself, "Will this matter in another 12 months? In 5 years?" This technique can quickly place things in a broader perspective.

Practice Self-Affirmation

A helpful method for decreasing test stress is to practice self-affirmation. After you have adequately studied and really know the material, stop and look in the mirror each time you pass one and say to yourself—preferably out loud—"I know this material, and I will do well on the test." After several times of watching and hearing yourself reaffirm your knowledge, you will gain inner confidence and be able to perform much better during the test period. This technique really works for students who are adventurous enough to use it. It may feel silly at first, but if it works, who cares? It will work for performing skills in clinical as well, as long as you have practiced the skill sufficiently.

Become More Assertive

Learn to stand up for your rights without violating the rights of others. Do not let people "walk all over you," because that leads to frustration, anger, and stress. Assertive techniques take practice, but a school counselor can help you get started. You will learn to show understanding of the other person's feelings but be able to assertively state what you need. Assertiveness is essential to becoming a patient advocate. See Chapter 6 for Internet resources on assertiveness.

Find Humor

Laughter is a great stress reliever. Watching a short program that makes you laugh, reading something funny, or sharing humor with friends helps decrease stress. Sometimes just putting a humorous twist on something that you are finding stressful relieves the stressed feeling. If you can manage to laugh many times a day, your stress levels should fall.

Refuel and Recharge

The old standbys of enough sleep and adequate nutritional intake also help keep excessive stress at bay. Although nursing students learn about the body's energy needs in anatomy and physiology classes, somehow they tend to forget that glucose is necessary for brain cells to work. Skipping breakfast or lunch or surviving on junk food puts the brain at a disadvantage. How can you expect to grasp material while reading textbooks if your brain is operating in a glucose-deficient mode? Can you perform in a top-notch manner in the clinical setting if the last meal was more than 8 hours ago? A car is not expected to run without gas; why should a body, and especially a brain, be expected to perform correctly when there is no fuel on board?

Once nursing classes start you will probably not be able to obtain the same amount of sleep as you did before, but rest is essential to the body and brain for good performance. Think of it as recharging the battery. A run-down battery provides only substandard performance. For most students, it is better to spend 7 hours sleeping and 3 hours studying than to cut sleep to 6 hours and study 4 hours. The improvement in the rested mind's efficiency will balance out the difference in the time spent studying. Knowing your natural body rhythms is necessary when it comes to determining the amount of sleep needed for personal learning efficiency.

Know Your Internal Clock

Determine whether you are a "lark" or an "owl." Larks, day people, do best getting up early and studying during daylight hours. Owls, night people, are more alert after dark and can remain up late at night studying, catching up on needed sleep during daylight hours. It is better to work with natural biorhythms than to try to conform to an arbitrary schedule. You will absorb material more quickly and retain it better if you use your most alert periods of each day for study. Of course, it is necessary to work around class and clinical schedules. Owls should attempt to register in afternoon or evening classes and clinical sections; larks do better with morning classes and day clinical sections.

Other Stress Remedies

- Take a walk.
- Play with a pet.
- Sit quietly and contemplate nature.
- Get a shoulder, back, or foot massage.
- Take a hot bath or shower.
- Talk out a stressful situation with a close friend.
- Write your thoughts and feelings in a journal.

■ STRESSES UNIQUE TO NURSING

Danger of Infection

Becoming a nursing student brings special situations that many find very stressful. Patients do not always get well; sometimes they die or lose body functions, an event that causes students considerable grief. Nurses care for patients with chronic or terminal diseases. Many diseases patients have can be contracted by the nurse. The following paragraphs present some information and suggestions for decreasing the fear of contracting harmful diseases and for dealing with dying patients.

PREVENTING CONTRACTION OF DISEASE

All health facilities have instituted the use of Standard Precautions to prevent health care workers from contracting harmful organisms through patient contact. The goal of Standard Precautions is to establish a barrier between the patient and anything that may transmit organisms to the worker or others. Personal protective equipment (PPE) such as vinyl or latex gloves, masks, gowns, and goggles are used when exposure to pathogenic organisms or body fluids that may contain human immunodeficiency virus (HIV) or hepatitis B or C virus is possible. Because it is not known which patients may harbor these harmful agents, all patients are considered to be potential carriers, and Standard Precautions are used for every patient. Gloves are used while working with patients when there is any chance of coming into contact with blood, other body fluids, and secretions (except sweat). Dressings and linens may be contaminated, and you should wear gloves when handling these items. Box 3-1 presents a synopsis of the Centers for Disease Control and Prevention's Standard Precautions.

BASIC SELF-PROTECTION

Self-protection against all disease is provided by following all infection control guidelines within the clinical facility. *Good hand hygiene* is the most effective method of reducing transfer of microorganisms from one person or object to another. Getting into the habit of washing hands or using hand sanitizer after each patient contact, before gloving, and when you remove gloves is one way to help decrease fear of contracting harmful organisms.

It is preferable to use nitrile rather than latex gloves because many people develop an allergy to latex.

Several drug-resistant microorganisms are encountered in the hospital and the community. Methicillin-resistant *Staphylococcus aureus* (MRSA) and vancomycin-resistant enterococci (VRE), as well as the *Clostridium difficile* organism, can cause very serious infections. Strictly adhering to Standard Precautions at work and practicing good asepsis at home and in the community setting will protect you.

WORKING WITH PATIENTS WITH AIDS

Developing an understanding of HIV and how it is transmitted is primary for decreasing the stress of working with the patient with HIV/AIDS. Adhering to Standard Precautions is all that is necessary when you have direct patient contact. Focus on the patient with HIV as a person with needs just like any other patient. Remembering to think through a procedure carefully before beginning it will help you use proper barrier precautions, such as gloves, goggles, mask, and gown, when needed. Whenever working with needles or other sharp objects, remember to move slowly and carefully to prevent sticks. When working with an individual known to be HIV positive and when blood contact is probable, use either a double-gloving technique if gloves are vinyl or use high-quality latex gloves. Never assume that blood will not splash inadvertently into your eyes or mouth, touching your mucous membranes. It is better to wear goggles and a mask than to be directly exposed to the virus.

Keeping the immune system in top functioning order should be another priority for every nursing student and nurse. This is accomplished by getting sufficient sleep, eating properly balanced meals, exercising regularly, attending to minor illnesses quickly, and keeping stress levels within limits. Along with the use of Standard Precautions, boosting the immune system is the best protection against HIV.

As for the stress of working with all the problems that HIV patients often have, you must study the disease and the multiple system problems it causes. Skillful care, good assessment, and therapeutic communication are essential components of providing the patient with HIV/AIDS with compassionate, comprehensive nursing care.

Standard Precautions

BOX 3-1

Human immunodeficiency virus (HIV), the virus that causes acquired immunodeficiency syndrome (AIDS), can be transmitted through exposure to infected blood or blood components and certain body fluids. Currently, there is no cure for AIDS and no immunization against it. The increasing prevalence of this disease increases the risk that health care workers will be exposed to blood from patients infected with HIV. The Centers for Disease Control and Prevention (CDC) recommends using Standard Precautions, formerly known as Standard Blood and Body Fluid Precautions, for the care of all patients. These precautions are directed at preventing parenteral, mucous membrane, and nonintact skin exposures of health care workers to blood-borne pathogens such as HIV, hepatitis B virus (HBV), and hepatitis C virus (HCV). Because HBV and HCV cause serious illness (chronic hepatitis) and are known to predispose the patient to cancer of the liver, immunization with HBV vaccine is recommended as an important adjunct to Standard Precautions for health care workers who may be exposed to blood. There is no vaccine for hepatitis C. Other infection control measures are used in addition to Standard Precautions. The following is a summary of the CDC guidelines.

BODY FLUIDS

Use Standard Precautions for all body fluids and tissues. Blood is the single most important source of HIV, HBV, HCV, and other blood-borne pathogens in the health care facility. Standard Precautions are used in the presence of feces, nasal secretions, sputum, tears, urine, and vomitus. General infection control measures apply to the handling of these body fluids. Proper hand hygiene is mandatory.

GENERAL PRECAUTIONS

1. Use Standard Precautions for all patients.
2. Routinely use appropriate barrier precautions when contact with blood or other body fluids of any patient is anticipated.
   - Do not reuse gloves.
   - Do not wash or disinfect surgical or examination gloves for reuse.
3. Take precautions to prevent injuries caused by needles, scalpels, and other sharp instruments or devices during procedures; when cleaning used instruments; when disposing of used needles; and when handling sharp instruments after procedures.
   - Discard needle units uncapped and unbroken after use.
   - Place disposable syringes and needles, scalpel blades, and other sharp items in puncture-resistant containers.
   - Place puncture-resistant containers as close as practical to the areas in which sharp items are used.
4. Although saliva has not been implicated in the transmission of HIV infection, a barrier should be used for mouth-to-mouth resuscitation, or a resuscitation bag should be used. Mouthpiece barriers, resuscitation bags, or both should be available for use in areas in which the need for frequent resuscitation is probable, such as the emergency department.

HAND HYGIENE

Hand hygiene is the hallmark of preventing the spread of infectious organisms. The CDC has recently modified the hand hygiene guidelines.

- Wash the hands with a nonantimicrobial soap and water or an antimicrobial soap and water any time they are visibly soiled, contaminated with proteinaceous material, or visibly soiled with blood or body fluids.

Continued

Standard Precautions (cont'd)

- An approved alcohol-based hand rub may be used for hand hygiene when hands are not visibly soiled.
- Perform hand hygiene after touching blood, body fluids, secretions, excretions, and contaminated items even if gloves were worn.
- Perform hand hygiene immediately after removing gloves.
- Perform hand hygiene between patient contacts and when otherwise indicated to avoid transferring microorganisms to other patients or environments.
- Perform hand hygiene after handling potentially contaminated items.
- Perform hand hygiene between tasks and procedures on one body area before moving to another body area on the same patient to prevent cross-contamination of different body sites.
- Wash hands with nonantimicrobial soap and water or with antimicrobial soap and water if contact with spores (e.g., *Clostridium difficile* or *Bacillus anthracis*) is likely to have occurred. Alcohols, chlorhexidine, iodophors, and other antiseptic agents have poor activity against spores.
- Do not wear artificial fingernails or extenders when providing direct patient contact for patients at high risk for infection and associated adverse outcomes.
- Use appropriate barrier methods gloves, surgical mask, protective eyewear, face shield, gown, and apron—when participating in invasive procedures.

USE OF PERSONAL PROTECTIVE EQUIPMENT
- Wear appropriate personal protective equipment (PPE) when the nature of the patient contact indicates that contact with blood or body fluids may occur.
- Wear gloves when touching blood and body fluids, mucous membranes, or nonintact skin, or when handling items or surfaces soiled with blood or body fluids. When performing skin sticks such as injections, finger or heel sticks, venipuncture, and other vascular access procedures, use latex or other nonpermeable gloves.
- Change gloves after contact with each patient, and perform hand hygiene.
- Change gloves during patient care if the hands will move from a contaminated body site (e.g., perineal or wound area) to a clean body site.
- Wear impermeable gowns or aprons during procedures that are likely to generate splashes of blood or other body fluids.
- Wear masks and protective eyewear or face shields during procedures that are likely to generate drops of blood or other body fluids to prevent exposure of mucous membranes of the mouth, nose, and eyes.
- Wear a gown for direct patient contact if the patient has uncontained secretions or excretions; do not reuse gowns.
- Prevent contamination of clothing and skin during the process of removing PPE.
- When performing or assisting in a delivery, wear gloves and a gown when handling the placenta or the infant until blood and amniotic fluid have been removed from the infant's skin, and use gloves during post-delivery care of the umbilical cord.
- If a needle stick occurs through a glove or a glove becomes torn, remove it and don a new glove as quickly as patient safety permits.

SAFE INJECTION PRACTICES
- Use aseptic technique to avoid contamination of sterile injection equipment.
- Never reuse a syringe or needle after entering a patient's skin; never reuse a cannula or an intravenous (IV) connection.
- Use single-dose vials for parenteral medications whenever possible.

Continued

Standard Precautions (cont'd)

- If a multiple-dose vial must be used, both the needle and the syringe used to access the vial must be sterile.
- Do not use bags or bottles of IV solution as a common source of supply for multiple patients.

RESPIRATORY HYGIENE AND COUGH ETIQUETTE

- Cover the mouth and nose when sneezing or coughing, preferably coughing or sneezing into the crook of the elbow rather than into the hands.
- Use a mask when in patient care areas if a respiratory problem is causing a runny nose, coughing, or sneezing.
- Perform hand hygiene when hands have been in contact with respiratory secretions or have used tissues.

ENVIRONMENTAL CONSIDERATIONS

- Standard sterilization and disinfection procedures currently recommended for use in health care settings are adequate.
- Sterilize instruments or devices that enter sterile tissue or the vascular system before reuse.
- Clean and remove soiled areas on walls, floors, and other surfaces routinely; extraordinary attempts to disinfect or sterilize are not necessary.
- Use chemical germicides approved as hospital disinfectants and tuberculocides to decontaminate spills of blood and other body fluids. In the absence of a commercial germicide, a solution of sodium hypochlorite (i.e., household bleach) in a 1:10 dilution is effective.

PRECAUTIONS WITH SOILED LINENS

- Handle soiled linen as little as possible and with minimum agitation to prevent gross microbial contamination of the air and of persons handling the linen.
- Place linen soiled with blood or body fluids in leak-resistant biohazard bags at the location at which it was used.

HANDLING SPECIMENS

- Place all specimens of blood and listed body fluids in well-constructed containers with secure lids to prevent leakage during transport; place specimens in a marked biohazard bag.
- Be careful not to contaminate the outside of the container when collecting specimens.

INFECTIVE WASTE DISPOSAL

- Incinerate or autoclave infective waste before disposal in a sanitary landfill.
- Dispose of containers of secretions as biohazardous waste in specially marked bags or containers.

Adapted from Siegel JD, Rhinehart E, Jackson M, et al: *Guideline for isolation precautions: preventing transmission of infectious agents in healthcare settings 2007,* Atlanta, 2007, Centers for Disease Control and Prevention, Healthcare Infection Control Practices Advisory Committee.

Working with Patients Who Are Dying

First experiences with patients who are dying are very stressful for most students. Prepare yourself by knowing what you can do to help the patient. Be familiar with the stages of grief and dying, while realizing that each patient deals with impending death individually. The nurse's role is to provide basic care for and comfort to the patient. Attend to small tasks such as lubricating lips, straightening linen, offering a back rub or a foot rub, straightening the environment, making certain enough warmth is provided, and offering sips of fluid, for example. Provide adequate pain relief and provide comfort measures. Check with the patient about what he or she desires.

Psychologically, assist the patient through the stages of the coping process; help the patient face issues as honestly as possible by being supportive. All you need to do in this area is to let the patient know that you are available to talk about whatever is pertinent. Never force a subject on the patient. Be honest and ask questions cautiously about what the patient knows and feels. Take cues from the patient about what topics are acceptable to explore. Do not avoid the issues of the illness, complications, or impending death. The patient may need to talk to someone not personally involved.

Sometimes it is helpful to reminisce with the patient, going through his or her life and remembering the major landmarks and fun times. Encourage family members or significant others to remember the past with the patient as well. Best of all, just offer yourself by simply being there for the patient. Check his or her needs often, and offer to just sit quietly in the room as time permits.

Discuss any fears you have with your instructor. Be specific about questioning what to do in certain situations. Know what to expect with a particular patient as death approaches. Will breathing become labored? Will the skin become mottled? Will the patient become unconscious? Ask the nurse who is caring for the patient about the probable course for this patient. Knowing what to expect can greatly decrease your fear of the actual event. Also clarify your role in the event that the patient stops breathing or has a cardiac arrest. Usually you should stay with the patient and use the call system to call out for the primary nurse or charge nurse. Always determine whether the patient has a do-not-resuscitate (DNR) order. **If such an order has not been written, you must begin cardiopulmonary resuscitation as soon as a respiratory or cardiac arrest is observed, even though it is known that the patient is terminally ill.**

High Acuity Level Patients

The pace in acute care settings is fast, and patients in the hospital are much sicker than 20 years ago. The acuity level is often quite high, and patients have multiple problems, lines, tubes, and equipment in use as well as numerous medications to be administered. The best way to decrease the stress when assigned such patients, or multiple patients, is to stay focused on each patient and to be well prepared. Learn to anticipate possible patient events, such as deteriorating condition, infiltrated IV site, and complications common to the disorder.

Special Patient Situations

Being prepared to deal with patients who are depressed, hostile, aggressive, or manipulative can also help decrease stress on clinical days. Your nursing texts tell you how to determine whether a patient is depressed or manipulative, but you will probably be able to pick out hostile and aggressive patient behaviors through your own life experiences.

DEPRESSED PATIENTS
Nursing interventions that sometimes help depressed patients include the following:

- Quietly sit with the patient.
- Encourage performance of activities of daily living; assist as needed.

- Work slowly; be patient and gentle.
- Point out the patient's strengths and accomplishments; emphasize good qualities.
- Do not admonish the patient to "cheer up and look at the bright side of things"; do not be overly bright and cheerful.
- Encourage social interaction, particularly exercise.
- Be alert for signs of self-destruction and the potential for suicide.

Patients who are diagnosed with depression upon entry to the hospital must be screened for suicide risk. To screen for suicide risk, watch for the following:

- Signs of acute depression, excessive anxiety, delirium, or dementia
- Intoxication with alcohol or drugs or medical or psychological problems that have a significant impact on judgment
- History of chronic pain, chronic illness, or terminal cancer

Report findings indicating risk to your charge nurse and instructor.

MANIPULATIVE PATIENTS

Manipulative patients use a variety of means to get what they want from the nurse. This behavior has various causes. It may be the way the patient has learned to communicate or respond to stress; often the patient simply fears losing control. Some specific nursing interventions useful in dealing with the manipulative patient include the following:

- Respond to the inappropriate behavior as calmly as possible; set limits. If the patient is shouting, explain that shouting is inappropriate, is disturbing to other patients, and makes it impossible to help. Say, "Please stop shouting, and tell me how I can help you."
- Be consistent and firm. State *how often* you can check on him or her; restate this information as needed when a demand is made between scheduled times.
- Do not become defensive; do your best not to take insults personally. Establish a personal emotional distance but not a professional distance.
- Be aware of how this behavior affects you. The patient may remind you of previous experiences with manipulative family members or friends.
- When all else fails or if you get into a loud exchange indicating demanding behavior, tell the patient you are leaving the room because of his or her behavior and that you will be back when he or she has calmed down. State when you will be back, and then arrive on time.

HOSTILE PATIENTS

Hostile, aggressive behavior includes verbal or physical threats. This type of behavior is usually an attempt to maintain control over the situation. When another person becomes aggressive, the usual response is to become defensive. At times, aggressive behavior occurs in family members as well as in patients. Some helpful nursing interventions to use when these behaviors occur include the following:

- Let the person know you are aware of his or her anger; allow feelings to be expressed freely. Ask what is upsetting the person and inquire what can be done to help him or her feel less angry and frustrated. *Actively* listen. Do not place blame.
- Provide the opportunity for the patient to make suggestions about self-care; give in to demands that are not unreasonable.

- Encourage as much physical activity as possible to help release pent-up feelings.
- Allow the patient to make decisions and choices regarding his or her care or the timing of procedures and tasks of daily living. This provides a sense of power and control.
- Rather than responding to the content of what the person is ranting about, attempt to respond to the underlying feelings.
- When a patient raises his or her voice, lower yours. Treat the person as an adult.
- Do not make promises that cannot be kept. This destroys trust.
- Protect your safety if a situation escalates by taking the following actions:
- Maintain a safe distance from the patient while verbally interacting (at least an arm and a half's length away); maintain eye contact.
- Position yourself between the patient and the exit; keep your hands in sight.
- Remove potential weapons from the patient's reach; remove any item from around your neck.
- Know how to summon help.

THE PATIENT WHO HAS DIFFICULTY COMMUNICATING VERBALLY

You may find it stressful to be assigned to care for a patient who is aphasic and has difficulty communicating as a result of disease or brain injury from a stroke or head trauma. There are several different varieties of aphasia (e.g., expressive, receptive, global, mixed), and patients can experience the problem from a slight to a profound degree. Your nursing texts can give you specific suggestions for dealing with individual types of aphasia, but here are some general guidelines:

- Keep the environment as relaxed and quiet as possible.
- Assume that the patient can understand what is heard even though his or her speech is jargon (nonsensical) or the patient is mute.
- Speak to the patient on an adult level; do not treat the patient as mentally incompetent.
- Talk to the patient, not about the patient to someone else in the room.
- Face the patient, establish eye contact, and speak slowly and distinctly without dropping your voice level at the end of sentences. Do not shout.
- Give short, simple directions; use pantomime and body language to enhance the words.
- Phrase questions so that they can be answered with a yes or no, and look for nonverbal behavior that agrees with the patient's answer.
- Give the person time to respond to questions; processing may be slower than usual.
- Do not ask more than one question at a time.
- If there is a need to repeat something, use the same words the second time. If difficulty still exists, phrase what was said differently.
- Allow only one person to speak at a time.
- Be very patient.

Remember that the person may get very frustrated when unable to verbalize adequately. A statement such as, "It must be very difficult and frustrating not to be able to make people understand what you want to say" and a caring touch may help. An understanding of what it must be like for the person may help keep you from becoming short and impatient. Be aware that aphasia worsens with anxiety or fatigue.

Personal Safety

Nurses often work shift hours and must travel in the dark. General safety rules for driving and walking, such as these, should be followed:

- Keep car doors locked at all times.
- Look in the back seat before entering the car.
- Have the car door key or release out and ready before you depart from the building.
- Be certain to keep the gas tank at least one quarter full at all times. Keep the car in good running condition.
- Travel on well-lighted, busy streets, avoiding isolated back roads and troubled parts of town.
- If you are being followed, drive to the nearest open business for help or drive to a police or fire station.
- Park only in areas that are well lighted. When leaving the clinical facility, walk with several other people or ask the security guard to accompany you during early morning or nighttime hours.
- Do not stop to aid a stranger in a stalled vehicle; proceed to an open business and report the stalled vehicle to the police.
- If you have vehicle trouble, raise the hood, get back into your vehicle, and lock it. Turn on the flashers. When someone offers assistance, roll down the window only enough to talk, and ask the person to call a relative, friend, garage, or the police for you. Never get into a stranger's car.
- Avoid walking alone. When you walk, do not keep looking down; walk with your head up and shoulders back, and survey your surroundings; make eye contact with passersby.
- Stay in well-lighted, pedestrian-traveled areas. Avoid shortcuts through alleys, parks, vacant lots, and deserted areas.
- If someone stops and asks for directions, maintain your distance; especially, do not approach a stopped car.
- If you are being followed, briskly walk to the nearest business or residence for help.
- If you are bothered by people in a car, turn and walk the other way.
- Women should hold a purse close and securely; avoid carrying extra money and valuables.
- Have your door key ready before leaving your car to enter your home.
- Be alert; note the people around you, your surroundings, and the total environment.

RAPE PREVENTION AND RESPONSE

Classes in personal defense for women are offered at most colleges and in many communities. A few hours spent learning methods of self-defense can prevent injury or rape. Following the preceding safety tips when walking and driving also can help prevent rape. However, should you be threatened with rape, there are some things that may prevent its occurrence. Active resistance is one way, and it must be used quickly. The purpose is to startle or surprise your attacker. For active resistance, use whatever you have as a weapon. Kick, use your elbow, scream, yell, or run; use your keys, purse, or whatever you have. A spray device with mace, tear gas, or pepper is effective, and nurses or students who have to walk to distant parking lots would be wise to have such a device in hand before leaving the building. Most such devices attach to a key ring.

Should rape occur, call the police *immediately*. In addition, call the local rape crisis center for quick counseling and a support person. It is important *not* to take a bath or shower. Physical evidence, including seminal fluid, hairs, scrapings of flesh from under fingernails, and any of the attacker's blood on the victim, is necessary for positive identification of the attacker and a court conviction. The police will ask for information about the car the attacker was driving, including make, color, and license plate number; the attacker's race, approximate age, weight, height, color and length of hair, and color of eyes; clothing the attacker was wearing, including hat, tie, shirt, pants, shoes, and glasses; and any unusual marks, scars, tattoos, piercings, or rings. Knowing whether the attacker is right handed or left handed is also helpful.

■ SELF-ASSESSMENT

Assessing Your Stress Level

Sometimes no matter what stress reduction techniques are used, the stresses of keeping up with classes, clinical, family, and job can become too much. Keep a finger on the pulse of your stress by assessing your stress status about once a month. Ask the following questions:

- Are you easily angered by uncontrollable events such as being put on hold on the telephone, traffic jams, persistent poor weather patterns, or malfunctioning equipment?
- Do you feel rushed all the time because tasks seem to never end?
- Has your sleep pattern changed? Do you have difficulty falling or staying asleep?
- Has your eating pattern changed? Have you lost or gained weight?
- Are you tired, anxious, or feeling "burned out" all the time?
- Do you suffer from chronic headaches, backaches, stiff neck or shoulder, or intestinal or stomach complaints?
- Do you often find yourself clenching or grinding your teeth?
- Are you drinking or smoking more than usual?
- Do you often lose your temper or burst into tears without a good reason?
- Are you constantly irritable?

Addressing Your Stress

If the answer is "yes" to three or more of the preceding questions, sit down and evaluate how you can decrease the stress levels in your life. If you do not believe you can change anything, seek professional assistance. Counseling is available at your school, from instructors, school counselors, and the school health center. You pay for these services when you register for your classes, so use them. Do not wait to go for help. The quicker you resolve the problem, the better your chance for success in school.

Using a relaxation technique will help you keep stress levels under control. However, to be useful, the technique must be used regularly several times a week until using it becomes second nature (Boxes 3-2 and 3-3).

Guided Imagery for Relaxation

BOX 3-2

This is a sample script for a guided imagery experience. It can be recorded and replayed while doing the exercise. Writing your own script and recording it maximizes the experience. When recording your script, read slowly in a soft but audible voice. Pause sufficiently after each instruction and section to allow time for following the instruction or forming the mental image. Performing this guided imagery exercise regularly can reduce stress.

When performing the exercise, sit or lie down and stretch out. Reduce noise and other distractions as much as possible. Dimming the light in the room is beneficial.

SCRIPT

- Close your eyes and gently relax.
- Take a deep, slow breath. Feel your lungs fill with clean, fresh air. Slowly exhale, sending all tension out with the air you exhale.
- Take another deep, slow breath; let it out slowly, sending body tension with it.
- Visualize yourself walking on a path in the woods at the edge of a meadow.
- Smell the clean air, the forest, and the flowers in the meadow.
- Feel the warmth of the sun and the soft, warm breeze. Hear the crunch of pine needles under your feet. It is so peaceful and serene here.
- You approach a brook, gently gurgling over the rocks in its path. You listen to the pleasant sound of the running water. It is almost as if the brook talks to you, welcoming you to this beautiful place of peace, comfort, and serenity.
- You look at the grass and moss growing in beautiful greens beneath the water.
- Patches of sunlight filtering through the trees warm your body. What a perfect spot to enjoy.
- You find a comfortable place, spread the blanket you were carrying, and sit and gaze at the trees, the meadow, and the blue sky with fluffy white clouds slowly moving to the horizon. What a beautiful place.
- You listen to the birds calling to each other and contemplate their cheerful melodies.
- A butterfly flits across your field of vision. You watch it as it zigzags across the meadow, going from flower to flower.
- It is so warm, pleasant, and peaceful here. You remember other days in similar surroundings.
- You concentrate on the feelings of warmth and peace the sun and breeze convey to you. Happiness fills your heart and soul, and you realize you can return here anytime you wish. This place is yours.
- Replenished, you arise, fold the blanket, and prepare to return up the path.
- You look around you once more—at the trees, the meadow, the sky, and the brook—imprinting the scene in your memory to take with you. This is your special place; it will always be here for you.
- You walk slowly up the path through the sunlight toward home.
- When you are ready, open your eyes.

Relaxation Exercise

BOX 3-3

This exercise is performed by recording the following script onto audiotape or an MP3 player and following the instructions as it is played. Using the exercise regularly over a period of weeks makes it easier to call on these techniques to induce relaxation during an exam or at other times you feel particularly tense.

Slowly read the script in a soft, firm voice. Allow sufficient pauses between segments for the instructions to be followed. Sit in a chair or lie down to do the exercise. Decrease outside noise and distractions as much as possible.

SCRIPT

- Close your eyes and find something to focus on mentally. It may be a spot of light, your pulse, a visual image, or whatever you choose. Try to hold it constant.
- Breathe in slowly and deeply; hold it a moment, and slowly breathe out. Now breathe normally, slowly, in and out.
- Tighten the muscles in your face and neck as firmly as you can, while clenching your teeth. Feel the tension. Hold it; slowly relax the muscles. Feel the relaxation in your face, jaw, and neck.
- With less tension, tighten the muscles in the face, jaw, and neck again. Feel this level of tension. Let go and relax. Notice the feeling of relaxation.
- Tighten the muscles in your chest firmly. Hold it; feel the tension. Let the chest muscles relax. Notice the difference between the tension and relaxation.
- With less tension, tighten the chest muscles again. Now let the muscles relax. Feel the relaxation.
- Tighten the fists and arm muscles as hard as possible. Hold the tension a moment. Slowly relax the muscles. Notice the difference in feeling between tension and relaxation.
- With less tension, tighten the fists and arm muscles again. Hold it. Let the muscles relax. Feel the relaxation.
- Tighten the abdominal muscles firmly. Hold the tension, noting the feeling. Relax the muscles, noting the difference between tension and relaxation.
- With less tension, tighten the abdominal muscles again. Hold it. Allow the muscles to relax completely. Notice the feeling of relaxation.
- Tighten the muscles in your right leg and foot. Hold the tension. Note the feeling. Allow the muscles to relax. Notice the difference between tension and relaxation.
- With less tension, tighten the muscles in your right leg and foot again. Hold it. Completely let go of the tension in the muscles and relax. Feel the relaxation.
- Tighten the muscles in your left leg and foot firmly. Hold it. Note the tension. Allow the muscles to relax. Focus on the difference between tension and relaxation.
- With less tension, tighten the muscles in your left leg and foot again. Hold it. Completely let go of the tension in the muscles and relax. Notice the feeling of relaxation.
- Breathe in and out deeply and slowly five times, focusing on your breathing.
- When you are ready, open your eyes.

4 CONTINUING YOUR EDUCATION

■ TAKING THE NEXT STEP

Types of Programs

Some colleges offer a ladder program within the nursing division. Some programs begin with a certified nursing assistant (CNA) curriculum that progresses to a 1-year practical nurse program. When this 1-year program is completed, the student has the option to complete a second year for an Associate Degree in Nursing (ADN) or continue for a Bachelor of Science in Nursing (BSN).

A number of colleges and universities offer a BSN completion program for ADN graduates. In these programs it generally takes 1 to $1\frac{1}{2}$ years to complete the nursing part of the curriculum. The completion program can be accomplished via online and distance learning. Today many colleges and universities offer online learning, condensed programs, and many other options for varied student needs.

Traditional BSN programs require 4 to 5 years to complete. These programs usually provide a more rounded education with required courses in the arts and sciences. The nursing courses usually do not begin until after the first 2 years of study. Students who are already licensed nurses may receive credit for some previous nursing courses. A master's degree in nursing (MSN) and a doctorate of nursing practice (DNP) can also be obtained by online and distance learning in many instances once a BSN has been earned. Some schools offer a BSN by online learning to graduates with degrees in other health-related fields.

The following four ways are available to evaluate an RN-to-BSN program or a BSN/MSN-to-DNP program:

1. Check the amount of general education units required. You should not have to repeat courses you have already successfully completed.
2. Look at the number of nursing courses required. Again, you should not have to repeat coursework you have already completed in a previous program.
3. Check the courses required and the amount of time required to earn the degree.
4. Calculate the entire cost of the program. Consider the cost of textbooks and any required travel.

Returning Students

Returning to school is a big step. If you have been in the workforce for many years, the student role will be a bigger adjustment for you than for those who recently graduated from a nursing program. The written work required for ADN, BSN, or BSN-completion programs is extensive, and a heavy emphasis is placed on the nursing process, concept-based learning, and evidence-based practice. You will review the nursing process during the first few weeks of class. Do your best to develop a good understanding of each component, how it works, and how the five parts are integrated with the application of the whole circular process. Spending time now to review the nursing process, especially as it relates to paperwork, will save you considerable time and frustration in your nursing classes and clinical courses. Explore how to research evidence-based nursing care.

Differences in Training

An even greater emphasis will be placed on the development and use of critical thinking throughout your nursing courses. If you graduated many years ago and have been working as a licensed nurse, studying critical thinking skills would be wise. Most fundamentals of nursing texts address this content. Several good books aimed particularly at critical thinking in nursing are available on the market. An example is *Critical Thinking and Clinical Judgment: A Practical Approach to Outcome-Focused Thinking*, 5th edition (2013), by Rosalinda Alfaro-LeFevre.

The RN student is expected to learn in-depth assessment skills. Emphasis will be placed on extensive history taking and skillful, thorough physical assessment. Compared with the licensed practical nurse/licensed vocational nurse (LPN/LVN), the RN is expected to develop even greater expertise in identifying problems and detecting complications and changes in a patient's condition. If it has been some time since you have used all your physical assessment techniques, practicing them on friends and relatives is the best way to brush up and improve your skills.

The BSN student studies more in-depth supervisory and management content than the ADN student. The BSN student is also trained in community health and research techniques. A course in statistics is usually required. Some BSN curricula require more science and mathematics courses as well.

Differences in Curriculum and Demands

Your ADN or BSN curriculum is similar to the previous nursing curriculum but more comprehensive. The volume of reading is time consuming, and much written work must be completed. Try to cut your work schedule to 20 hours a week or less. Aim for success from the beginning. If you have spare time and see that your class average is good after working part time for a while, you can slowly increase your work hours. Only rarely can students with family commitments be successful in an RN program while working full time. Many single students who do not have other obligations have difficulty keeping up with school if they try to work 40 hours per week. Students who are single parents often need to work more hours, but they are at a disadvantage because they are the only caregivers for their families, which seriously limits available study time. Relatives can sometimes be asked to take total charge of the children for several hours, thereby providing blocks of study time one or more times a week for the months you are in school.

Bringing Skills and Habits with You

Depending on where you have been working, you will have some advantages over new nursing students. If you have been working in a hospital or long-term care facility, you should be confident and competent with skills such as administering medications, catheterization, and nasogastric tube insertion. You should also have an advantage in that you are familiar with many prescription drugs.

Sometimes instructors prefer that a skill be performed differently from how you learned it years earlier. Protocols and ideas on the best way to do things change from time to time as new information emerges on evidence-based nursing. If you learned a procedure differently in your previous nursing courses, you may have to practice outside of class to learn to perform the skill in a new way.

If you have been working in home care and regularly using your assessment skills, you may have an advantage over other students in this area. You can function independently and make decisions, and you have developed good people skills and know how to adapt to various situations.

If you have been working in a long-term care facility, you are very familiar with the problems and needs of older adults and with the ways of efficiently caring for this population. For example, you know the techniques that are helpful in administering medications to the person who has a decreased ability to swallow, how to distract the patient who has decided not to do what you want him or her to do, and how to quickly clean up the bed and skin of a patient who is incontinent.

If you have years of experience in a surgical department, you are comfortable and confident with sterile techniques. You have an idea why the patient has postoperative pain and why joints and muscles are sore and stiff after a lengthy operation. You are familiar with the routine of assisting with a cardiac or respiratory arrest.

Catching up with Generic Students

Unless you work in an area in which you manage a variety of drugs, you will need to spend extra time refreshing your pharmacological knowledge when you enter an ADN or a BSN program. Generic students may have had many months to study drugs. You should start refreshing your memory about a set number of drugs each week from the first week. Learn the drugs first by classification and then by family group. If you understand how the class of drugs works, you can determine the possible side effects and then determine the probable nursing implications. After you have learned the classification information, choose individual drugs that differ in side effects or nursing implications from the general drugs of the class, and learn those.

One problem many returning students have is adopting the role of a student when they are in a clinical setting. Each student should clarify with the instructor which skills can be performed without supervision and which skills the instructor must be called on to observe. Although performing a procedure while working as a licensed nurse is so natural, as a student, you might easily forget that you simply cannot just do it. Get into the "think before doing" mode during your clinical experience hours.

Role Transformation

As you near the end of the RN curriculum, you will be learning more advanced supervision of others. Advanced leadership skills are part of the RN competencies. Sometimes a practical nurse who has little supervisory experience may find it difficult to act in a leadership role. One way to prepare for leadership is to observe continually how the charge nurse and staff RNs interact and delegate tasks to the other personnel on the unit. Role-play for yourself how you would handle various situations and assignments within your daily work routine. Observe the nuances of supervision in action.

The BSN student should begin to see the larger picture from the standpoint of administration and the institution. This perspective requires a broadened mindset. For an ADN, the focus is on providing patient care. For a BSN, the focus expands to include the needs of the nursing unit and the institution as well as the patient. Aspects of the new role include learning to schedule personnel, managing conflicts among staff, writing policies, and performing evaluations of staff. A greater emphasis is put on long-term quality improvement.

Try to mainstream yourself with all the students rather than segregating yourself with other returning practical nurses or ADNs. In this way you can glean information that other students learned during their courses for which you received credit because of your previous nursing classes. You can find out which instructors may suit your needs and personality the best, and you will have some assistance in refining your paperwork from those who have already been through some of the assignments. Share your expertise when asked; it will boost your morale. You have a lot to offer to the learning experience of the group.

Success begins with planning. Consistently using this planner for scheduling your time for study, exams, classes, and other activities can help you achieve success in the nursing program, whether you are a returning practical nurse, an ADN, or a beginning BSN student.

Continuing Your Education

■ COMMUNICATION

Prefixes and Suffixes Used in Medical Terms

Term	Meaning	Term	Meaning
Combining Forms		naso-	nose
adeno-	gland	nephro-	kidney
alveolo-	air sac	neuro-	nerve
andro-	man, male	onco-	mass, tumor
angio-	vessel	oophoro-	ovary
appendic/o-	appendix	ophthalmo-	eye
arthro-	joint	orchio-	testis
audio-	hearing	osteo-	bone
bio-	life	oto-	ear
broncho-	bronchus	patho-	disease
carcino-	cancerous	pharyngo-	pharynx
cardio-	heart	pneumo-	lung, air
ceco-	cecum	procto-	rectum, anus
cephalo-	head	prostato-	prostate
cerebro-	brain	psycho-	mind
cervico-	neck	pyelo-	kidney
chole-	bile	radi-	ray, radiation
cholecysto-	gallbladder	rhino-	nose
claviculo-	clavicle	salpingo-	tube
colo-	colon	spleno-	spleen
cranio-	skull	stoma-	mouth
cutaneo-	skin	thrombo-	clot
cysto-	bladder, sac	thyro-	thyroid
dermato-	skin	tracheo-	trachea
duodeno-	duodenum	tricho-	hair
encephalo-	brain	uretero-	ureter
entero-	intestine	uro-	urine
erythro-	red	vertebro-	vertebra
esophago-	esophagus	**Prefixes**	
gastro-	stomach	a-, an-	without, away from, not, no
gingivo-	gums	ab-	away from, absent
gluco-	sugar	ana-	up, back, again
gyneco-	woman	ante-	before
hemato-	blood	auto-	self
hepato-	liver	bi-	two, twice
hystero-	uterus	co-, con-	with, together
laryngo-	larynx	contra-	opposite, against
leuko-	white	dia-	through, complete
lipo-	fat	dys-	difficult, painful, abnormal
meningo-	membrane		
myelo-	marrow, spinal cord		
myo-	muscle		

Prefixes and Suffixes Used in Medical Terms (cont'd)

Term	Meaning	Term	Meaning
ec-, ecto-	outside, out	-iasis	morbid condition
endo-, ento-	within	-ic	pertaining to
epi-	above	-ist	one who specializes in
exo-	out		
hyper-	excessive, above	-itis	inflammation
hypo-	below, deficient	-logy	process of study
meta-	change, over, after	-lysis	dissolution, setting free
peri-	around, surrounding, about	-malacia	softening, soft
pro-	before, in front of	-megaly	enlargement
re-	back, again	-oid	form, shape
retro-	behind, backward	-ology	study or science of
sym-, syn-	together, with	-oma	tumor
trans-	across, through, beyond	-opsy	viewing
		-osis	condition, disease
		-pathy	disease, suffering
Suffixes		ponia	deficiency, lack of, decrease
-ac	pertaining to		
-al	pertaining to	-pexy	fixation
-algia	painful condition, pain	-plasty	mold, shape, repair
		-ptosis	downward displacement, falling
-cele	hernia, swelling, sac		
-centesis	puncture of a cavity	-rhea	flow, discharge
-cyte	cell	-scope	instrument to visually examine
-desis	fusion, binding, fixation	-scopy	process of examining
-ectasis	expansion, dilation	-sis	state of, condition
-ectomy	excision, removal of a body part	-spasm	involuntary spasm
		-stasis	control, constant level
-emia	blood		
-genic	origin, formation	-stomy	creation of an opening
-gram	the record made, mark	-therapy	treatment
		-tome	instrument for cutting
-graph	instrument for recording, machine	-tomy	process of cutting
		-trophy	nourishment
-graphy	the process, process of recording		
-ia	condition		

Adapted from O'Toole M, editor: *Dictionary of medicine, nursing, and health professions,* ed 9, St Louis, 2013, Mosby.

Commonly Used Abbreviations, Symbols, and Notations

Abbreviations

ad lib—as desired
ADLs—activities of daily living
AK—above the knee
AMA—against medical advice

amb—ambulate
ax—axillary
BP—blood pressure
BK—below the knee
C—centigrade

CABG—coronary artery bypass graft
CCU—cardiac care unit
CDC—Centers for Disease Control

Continued

Commonly Used Abbreviations, Symbols, and Notations (cont'd)

CMS—Centers for Medicare and Medicaid services

c/o—complains of

CPAP—continuous positive airway pressure

CPM—continuous passive motion

CPOE—computerized provider order entry

CPR—cardiopulmonary resuscitation

CXR—chest x-ray

dx—diagnosis

DNI—do not intubate

DNR—do not resuscitate

DOB—date of birth

DOE—dyspnea on exertion

DRG—diagnosis-related group

DTR—deep tendon reflex

ECT—electric convulsive therapy

ED—emergency department

EHR—electronic heath record

EMR—electronic medical record

EOM—extraocular movement

ESR—erythrocyte sedimentation rate

ETOH—alcohol

F—Fahrenheit

FBS—fasting blood sugar

FUO—fever of unknown origin

GB—gallbladder

GFR—glomerular filtration rate

GU—genitourinary

hr—hour

HIPAA—Health Insurance Portability and Accountability Act

HIT—health information technology

H&P—history and physical

HOB—head of bed

HOH—hard of hearing

hx—history

ICU—Intensive care unit

I&O—intake and output

IOP—intraocular pressure

KCl—potassium chloride

KUB—kidney, ureters, bladder

KVO—keep vein open

LBW—low birth weight

LE—lower extremity

LLE—left lower extremity

LLL—left lower lobe

LLQ—left lower quadrant

LUQ – left upper quadrant

LMP—last menstrual period

LOC—level/loss of consciousness

LP—lumbar puncture

LUE—left upper extremity

LUL—left upper lobe

NG—nasogastric

NPO—nothing by mouth

NV—nausea and vomiting

OOB—out of bed

ORIF—open reduction and internal fixation

OT—occupational therapy

P—pulse

PCA—patient-controlled analgesia

PDR—Physicians' Desk Reference

PERRLA—pupils equal, round, and reactive to light and accommodation

PICC—percutaneously inserted central catheter

PND—paroxysmal nocturnal dyspnea

PRN—as required (*pro re nata*)

PT—physical therapy

PVC—premature ventricular contraction

q—every

R—respirations

RDA—recommended daily allowance

RLE—right lower extremity

RLL—right lower lobe

RLQ—right lower quadrant

R/O—rule out

ROM—range of motion

RUE—right upper extremity

RUL—right upper lobe

RUQ—right upper quadrant

SS—social service

SNF—skilled nursing facility

SOB—shortness of breath

T—temperature

TCDB—turn, cough, and deep breathe

TED—thromboembolic disease

TENS—transcutaneous electrical stimulation

TM—tympanic membrane

TPN—total parenteral nutrition

TURP—transurethral resection of the prostate

tx—treatment

UA—urinalysis

VS—vital signs

VSD—ventral septal defect

WNL—within normal limits

wt—weight

×—times

Symbols

△—change

↑—increase, up

⊕—positive, present

↓—decrease, down

⊖—negative, not present

Medication Routes

IM—intramuscular

IV—intravenous

IVPB—intravenous piggyback

PO—by mouth

PR—by rectum

SL—sublingual

Subcut—subcutaneous

Commonly Used Abbreviations, Symbols, and Notations (cont'd)

Medication Frequency

AC—before meals
bid—twice a day

PC—after meals
PRN—as needed

qid—four times a day
tid—three times a day

Medications

ASA—aspirin
NSAIDs—nonsteroidal antiinflammatory drugs

Medication Dosages

g—gram
gr—grain
gtt—drops

L—liter
mcg, μg—microgram
mEq—milliequivalent

mg—milligram
mL—milliliter
tsp—teaspoon

Serum Laboratory Tests

C&S—culture and
  sensitivity
CBC—complete blood
  count
ESR—erythrocyte
  sedimentation rate
Hb, Hgb—hemoglobin

Hct—hematocrit
K^+—potassium
LFTs—liver function tests
Na^+—sodium
PSA—prostate-specific
  antigen

PT—prothrombin time
PTT—partial
  thromboplastin time
RBCs—red blood cells
WBCs—white blood cells

Other Terms

AO × 4—alert, oriented to
  person, place, date,
  and time or situation
c̄—with

C—cervical
CSF—cerebrospinal fluid
HA—headache
L—lumbar

MVA—motor vehicle
  accident
STAT—immediately
s̄—without

Diseases and Disorders

ALS—amyotrophic lateral
  sclerosis
AMI—acute myocardial
  infarction
ARDS—acute respiratory
  distress syndrome
BPH—benign prostatic
  hypertrophy
Ca—cancer
COPD—chronic obstructive
  pulmonary disease

CP—cerebral palsy
CVA—cerebrovascular
  accident
DKA—diabetic ketoacidosis
DM—diabetes mellitus
ESRD—end-stage renal
  disease
MS—multiple sclerosis
RA—rheumatoid arthritis
SLE—systemic lupus
  erythematosus

STI—sexually
  transmitted
  infection
TIA—transient ischemic
  attack
URI—upper respiratory
  infection
UTI—urinary tract infection

Diagnostic Tests

CAT or CT—computed
  axial tomography or
  computed tomography
ECG—electrocardiogram
EEG—electroencephalogram

EKG—electrocardiogram
EMG—electromyography
MRI—magnetic resonance
  imaging

PET—positron emission
  tomography

Adapted from O'Toole M, editor: *Dictionary of medicine, nursing, and health professions*, ed 9, St Louis, 2013, Mosby.

SBAR Communication Tool

The intent of the *SBAR* tool is to overcome communication barriers between doctors and nurses, between nurses, and between nurses and other health care professionals. It can help prevent care lapses and mistakes when the patient is handed off from one nurse to another or when the patient is transferred to another unit or facility. The acronym provides a quick and concise method of conveying detailed information in incident or emergency situations. The acronym stands for **S**ituation, **B**ackground, **A**ssessment, **R**ecommendation or **R**equest. Here is an example:

S: Dr. Savoy, this is Nurse Lopez at ABC Extended Care Facility. Mr. Tanglewood is an 85-year-old with Alzheimer's disease. He tripped in the bathroom and bumped his head on the toilet about 30 minutes ago. One of the nursing assistants saw him trip; there was no loss of consciousness at any time.

B: He is normally alert and oriented to person, and he routinely ambulates.

A: His blood pressure is 140/83, pulse 75, respirations 16 per min. He has a 3-cm laceration and hematoma just superior to his left eyebrow. The bleeding was readily controlled with direct pressure. We have applied an ice pack and pressure bandage over the wound. He is alert, and his speech is clear and appropriate to his baseline. He denies any pain, and he does not seem to have tenderness or bruising except on his forehead, but he did extend his right hand to break his fall.

R: Could I get an order to have him transported to the emergency department for additional evaluation and treatment? And do you have any additional orders for Mr. Tanglewood?

Adapted from deWit SC, O'Neill P: *Fundamental concepts and skills for nursing*, ed 4, Philadelphia, 2014, Saunders.

Basic Phrases in English and Spanish

Question or Phrase in English	Question or Phrase in Spanish	Phonetic Pronunciation
Do you speak English?	¿Habla usted inglés?	ah-blah oo-stehd een-glehs?
I don't understand.	No entiendo.	noh ehn-t-yehn-doh.
My name is...	Me llamo...	meh yah-moh...
What is your name?	¿Cuál es su nombre?	kwahl ez soo nom bray?
Speak more slowly, please.	Hable más despacio, por favor.	ah-bleh mahs deh-spah-see-yoh, pohr fah-vohr.
I'm here to help you.	Estoy aquí para ayudarle.	ehs-toy ah-kee pah-rah ah-yoo-dahr-leh.
I'm going to take your vital signs.	Le voy a tomar los signos vitales.	leh voy ah toh-mahr lohs seeg-nohs vee-tah-lehs.
I'm going to take your pulse.	Le voy a tomar el pulso.	leh voy ah toh-mahr ehl pool-soh.
I'm going to take your blood pressure.	Le voy a tomar la presión.	leh voy ah toh-mahr lah preh-syohn.
I'm going to take your temperature.	Le voy a tomar su temperatura.	leh voy ah toh-mahr soo tehm-peh-rah-too-rah.
Do you understand?	¿Entiende usted?	ehn-t-yehn-deh oo-stehd?
Are you allergic to anything?	¿Es usted alérgico(a) a cualquier cosa?	ehs oo-stehd ah-lehr-hee-koh(kah) ah kwahl-kee-yehr koh-sah?
Do you take any medications?	¿Toma medicamentos?	toh-mah meh-dee-kah-mehn-tohs?

Basic Phrases in English and Spanish (cont'd)

Question or Phrase in English	Question or Phrase in Spanish	Phonetic Pronunciation
Here is the call light.	Aquí está la luz para llamar a la enfermera.	ah-kee eh-stah lah looss pah-rah yah-mahr ah lah ehn-fehr-meh-rah.
This is the television control.	Este es el control de la televisión.	ehs-teh ehs ehl kohn-trohl deh lah teh-leh-vee-see-yohn.
This is the bed control.	Este es el control de la cama.	ehs-teh ehs ehl kohn-trohl deh lah kah-mah.
Don't get out of bed by yourself.	No se baje de la cama solo(a).	noh seh bah-heh deh lah kah-mah soh-loh(ah).
You may not eat or drink anything more before surgery.	No comerá o beberá nada antes de la cirujía.	Noh koh-meh-rah oh beh-beh-rah nah-dah ahn-tehs deh lah see-roo-hee-ah.
Do you have pain?	¿Tiene dolor?	t-yeh-neh doh-lohr?
Are you nauseated?	¿Siento el estómago revuelto?	s-ehn-teh ehl ehs-toh-mah-goh reh-vwehl-toh?
Take a deep breath in, please. Exhale.	Respire profundo, por favor. Exhale.	reh-spee-reh proh-foon-doh, pohr fah-vohr. ehks-ah-leh.
Now cough.	Ahora tosa.	ah-or-a toh-sah.
I am going to give you an injection.	Le voy a poner una inyección.	leh voy ah poh-nehr oo-nah een-yehk-see-yohn.
I have some medications for you to take.	Tengo unas medicamentos para que usted las tome.	tehn-goh oo-nahs meh-dee-kah-mehn-tohs pah-rah keh oo-steh id lahs toh-meh.
When was your last bowel movement?	¿Cuándo tuvo último excremento?	kwahn-doh too-voh soo ool-tee-moh ehks-kreh-mehn-toh?
I need to measure your urine.	Debo medir su orina.	day-bow meh-deer soo oh-ree-nah.
It is time for your bath.	Es hora de su baño.	ehs oh-rah deh soo bahn-yoh.
Do not pull on the tube.	No jale el tubo.	noh hah-leh el too-boh.
Sit up, please.	Siéntese, por favor.	s-yehn-teh-seh, pohr fav-vohr.

■ BASIC PRINCIPLES OF NURSING CARE

The Nursing Process

The five-step nursing process (pictured on the inside front cover) is set in motion at the time of the initial assessment. There is continuous interaction among the components, and the patient is the focus of all activities within the process. Arrows point in both directions, indicating that the process is always in motion. Thus each component is subject to revision as new information is obtained through interaction with the patient. Following are some examples of activities used within each step of the nursing process.

ASSESSMENT
- Data gathering
  - Initial admission assessment
  - Interview and history taking
  - Physical examination/assessment
  - Measure vital signs
  - Chart review
- Beginning of shift, quick head-to-toe assessment
- Focused assessment for major problem (e.g., respiratory, cardiac, neurologic)
- Assessment of equipment needed for a procedure
- Assessment of learning needs
- Review of literature
- Review of anatomy and physiology of body systems involved in patient problem
- Read about disease process or surgery
- Consult other health team members for further information

NURSING DIAGNOSIS
- Analysis of data to determine problem areas
- Definition of problems
- Formulation of problem statements/nursing diagnoses (RN)
- Recognition of appropriate nursing diagnoses chosen for care plan (LPN/LVN)
- Collaboration with patient for prioritization of problems/nursing diagnoses

PLANNING
- Write goals/expected outcomes for each problem.
- Set a time for expected outcomes to be met.
- Plan interventions to assist patient to meet expected outcomes or achieve goals.
- Devise a teaching plan.
- Check physician's orders to see what has to be done.
- Plan ahead for surgical care.
- Plan ahead for medication administration.
  - Check to see that medications are on the unit.
  - Verify medication orders on the medication administration record (MAR) with the physician's original orders.
- Collaborate with other health team members to plan patient's total care for the shift.
- Document the nursing care plan.
- Plan revision of interventions when evaluation indicates the need.
- Plan work organization for the shift.

IMPLEMENTATION
- Supervise implementation of the nursing care plan.
- Carry out planned nursing interventions.
- Delegate/assign tasks to ancillary nursing personnel.
- Perform skills and procedures.
  - Measure and record intake and output (I&O).
  - Change a dressing.

- Check equipment in use.
- Apply a heat treatment.
- Give medications.
- Teach patients.
- Counsel assigned patients and families.
- Consult/collaborate with other health team members (e.g., social worker, dietitian, pharmacist, physician).

EVALUATION
- Evaluate patient condition.
- Evaluate effect of nursing interventions.
- Determine whether nursing interventions are helping patient meet expected outcomes/goals.
- Evaluate data to see whether there is progress toward recovery.
- Evaluate whether interventions have to be revised.
- Evaluate effect of treatments.
- Evaluate for side effects and therapeutic effect of medications.
- Document evaluation data.
- Evaluate whether work organization schedule has to be revised.

Documentation
DESCRIPTIVE TERMS USED IN DOCUMENTATION

Word	Idea to Be Charted	Terms Suggested
Abdomen	Appearance	Distended, round, flat, soft, firm, hard, rigid, protruding, flaccid, tympanic, distended, tender, boardlike, bruised, or ecchymotic
Bleeding	In very large amounts or spurts	Spurting blood, profuse oozing
	Very little	Minimal amount; scant
	Location	Blood in vomitus (hematemesis), blood in urine (hematuria), blood in sputum, nosebleed (epistaxis), or black tarry stool (melena)
Breath	Taking air in	Inspiration
	Breathing air out	Expiration, exhalation
	Short time without breathing	Apnea
	Rapid breathing	Hyperpnea
	Cannot breathe lying down	Orthopnea
	Snoring sounds of breathing	Stertorous respiration
	Unpleasant odor	Halitosis
	Increasing dyspnea with periods of nonbreathing	Cheyne-Stokes respirations
	Difficulty breathing or labored breathing	Dyspnea
Convulsion	Muscles contract and relax	Clonic tremor or convulsion
	Muscle contraction maintained for a time	Tonic tremor or convulsion
	Localized muscle contraction	Spasm
	Begins without warning	Sudden onset
	Abrupt start and end of spasm or convulsive seizure	Paroxysm

DESCRIPTIVE TERMS USED IN DOCUMENTATION (cont'd)

Word	Idea to Be Charted	Terms Suggested
Cough	Various types of coughing	Tight, loose, deep, dry, hacking, painful, exhaustive, hollow
	Coughs all the time	Continuous
	Coughs over long period of time	Persistent
	Coughs up material	Productive
	Coughs without producing material	Nonproductive
	Sudden attacks of coughing	Paroxysmal
Consciousness	Aware of surroundings	Alert—conversant, fully awake, and conscious
	Partly conscious	Groggy, lethargic, semiconscious
	Arousable but not conscious; responds to some stimuli	Stuporous, semiconscious; responsive to verbal stimuli, responsive to tactile stimuli
	Unconscious, cannot be aroused; does not respond to stimuli	Comatose
Drainage	Water from the nose	Coryza
	Sticky	Viscous
	Bloody	Sanguineous
	Contains serum and blood	Serosanguineous
	Fecal (contains bowel material)	Fecal
	Contains mucus and pus	Mucopurulent
	From vagina after delivery	Lochia
Odor	Not pleasant; pungent	Aromatic
	Spicy like fruit	Fruity
	Unpleasant	Offensive; foul
	Smelling like a particular thing	Characteristic of...
Pain	Amount of pain	Use statement of patient; slight to severe; rate on a scale of 1 to 10
	Types of pain	Aching, dull, slight, burning, throbbing, gnawing, acute, chronic, generalized, superficial, excruciating, unyielding, cramping, darting, colicky, continuous, shifting, agonizing, piercing, intense, cutting, transient, localized, remittent, persistent
	Comes in seizures	Spasmodic
	Spreads to certain areas	Radiating
	Begins suddenly	Sudden onset
	Hurts when moving	Increased by movement
Skin	Terms to describe condition	Pale, pink, red, moist, dry, clear, coarse, tanned, scaly, thick, loose, rough, tight, infected, discolored, jaundiced, mottled, calloused, edematous, excoriated, abraded, bruised, painful, scarred, black, oily, yellow, brown, white, clammy, rash, wrinkled, smooth

DESCRIPTIVE TERMS USED IN DOCUMENTATION (cont'd)

Word	Idea to Be Charted	Terms Suggested
Speech	Unable to be understood	Incoherent
	Meaningless	Rambling, irrelevant
	Runs words together	Slurs
	Difficulty in speaking	Dysphasia
	Unable to speak	Aphasia
	Other terms to describe	Stammering, stuttering, hoarse, feeble, fluent, clear

HIPAA Considerations for Nurses

To follow the privacy rules outlined in the Health Insurance Portability and Accountability Act (HIPAA) and protect patients' privacy:

- Avoid discussion with patients about their condition within earshot of other patients or visitors. Use a low voice or take the patient to a private area for verbal interaction.
- Remove the patient record from the computer screen when you leave. Be certain that other patients or visitors cannot see the screen while you are working.
- Use only patients' initials on worksheets, assignment sheets, and student care plans and assignments.
- Do not discuss patients in the elevators, cafeteria, or other public locations, even with your same-unit personnel.
- Do not discuss patients with your family and friends at any time.
- Do not divulge patient information to patient's family or others without explicit patient permission.

Discharge

PATIENT TEACHING

Cover the following points when performing discharge teaching:
- Care of incision, if present
- Dressing changes, supplies, techniques, soiled dressing disposal
- Care of tubes, drain suction devices, other equipment in place
- Care of IV site
- Activity level permitted; restrictions
- When patient can return to work
- Driving restrictions
- Sexual activity guidelines
- Weight-lifting restrictions
- Bathing/showering precautions
- Rest requirements
- Diet guidelines; any restrictions
- Signs and symptoms to report
- When and where to make a follow-up appointment
- Medications, purpose, schedule, side effects to report
- Where to obtain medical equipment to be rented or purchased
- Number to call if questions arise

Clinical Quick Reference

WRITING A DISCHARGE SUMMARY

Follow your agency's format and guidelines regarding content. The following points are usually included in the discharge summary, which is written in the nurse's notes or on a discharge sheet or EMR flowsheet:

- Who received the teaching (patient, patient and family, family caregiver, etc.)
- A summary of the patient's care
- An outline of all patient teaching, including what the patient was taught about diagnosis, diet, activity, medications, wound care, special care, signs and symptoms of complications to report to the physician, use of medical equipment, follow-up care, and referrals
- Documentation that the patient understands the teaching and that written instructions have been given to him or her
- Any exceptional details or unusual findings regarding the illness or present condition
- Condition of the patient at the time of discharge
- Description of status of wounds, dressings, drains, and tubes still in place
- Where patient is told to call and the phone numbers should further help be needed

Standard Reference Materials

These references may be in book form on the units but are often online in the system computers or can be obtained by a mobile device app:

Drug reference: Contains information on drugs organized by generic name, brand name, or category of use. Use it to find pertinent information about drugs you will be giving.

Procedures manual/skills manual: Contains the accepted procedures for performing various nursing skills in the clinical facility. This thick book is an in-house volume and may vary in content from one clinical facility to another. Use it to review each nursing procedure before preparing to perform it (e.g., urinary catheterization, sterile dressing change).

Diet manual: Lists the foods allowed and forbidden on the various therapeutic diets available in the clinical facility. Use this manual to check what the patient may and may not have when a special diet is prescribed.

Documentation/charting manual: Designates the accepted procedures and forms to be used for documenting nursing care within the particular clinical facility. Use this manual to learn to correctly document the nursing care you give.

Medical dictionary: Provides definitions of medical terms, pronunciation of words, correct spelling of medical words, lists of abbreviations, and a variety of appendices that may include lists of symbols, prefixes and suffixes, nursing diagnoses, diagnosis-related groups (DRGs), tables of laboratory values, foreign language terms, anatomic tables or charts, food value charts, and other helpful aids.

Clinical nursing manual: Contains information about most procedures and patient conditions generally encountered by the average staff nurse.

General Steps for All Procedures

For all procedures, the following elements should be performed before the procedure is started:

- Check the physician's order.
- Obtain a signed consent form if required.

- Carry out any patient preparation necessary prior to the procedure.
- Gather equipment.
- Verify the patient's identity using name, ID number (possibly birth date). Obtain assistance if necessary (e.g., someone to hold patient).
- Provide privacy (e.g., close door, drape as appropriate).
- Explain the procedure to the patient.
- Obtain consent to proceed (verbal or implied for routine nursing procedures).
- Arrange work space as needed.
- Perform hand hygiene.

For all procedures, the following should be performed at the end of the procedure:

- Assess response to procedure (e.g., Does the catheter hurt?).
- Ensure safety; bed in low position (side rails up if needed).
- Rearrange environment for patient's convenience and comfort (call bell within reach).
- Thank patient and give any special instructions related to procedure.
- Dispose of equipment.
- Perform hand hygiene.
- Document procedure and patient response.

Guidelines for Cast Care

- Check the cast for integrity: no breaks, cracks, crumbling edges.
- Assess the degree of tightness around the casted part: it should not be cutting into the flesh.
- **Assess for circulation and movement distal to the cast: check pulses, skin temperature, ability to move joints, and sensation.**
- Assess for any pain related to the placement of the cast.
- Feel along the cast for "hot" spots that might indicate underlying infection.
- Smell the ends of the cast for any odor, which may indicate the presence of infection.
- Position the casted area per the physician's orders; support joints proximal and distal to the cast.
- Supervise range-of-motion exercises for joints proximal or distal to the cast as ordered.
- Caution patient not to poke anything under the cast.
- Handle a cast that is still wet with the flat of the palm of the hand rather than the fingertips when positioning.
- Listen to what the patient says and respond to any complaints with further exploration of the problem.

■ ASSESSMENT QUICK REFERENCE

Blood Pressure Parameters and Classifications

Classification	Systolic Measurement (mm Hg)		Diastolic Measurement (mm Hg)
Normal	<120	and	<80
Prehypertension	120-139	or	80-89
Stage I hypertension	140-159	or	90-99
Stage II hypertension	≥160	or	≥100

Neurologic Assessment

All patients should be routinely assessed for level of consciousness, orientation, and thought processes. Clinical facilities, especially long-term or psychiatric settings, are likely to have expanded versions of the mental status examination.

ORIENTATION AND MENTAL STATUS

Orientation
- What place is this?
- What is the date?
- What is your wife's maiden name?
- What is your husband's name?

Ability to follow simple instructions
- Hold out your left hand with the palm up.
- Please hand me the _____ (pen, pencil, book; providing free choice of several objects; also tests object recognition).

Memory
- Do you remember my name? (If so, what is it?)
- What did you have for breakfast this morning?

Delirium and dementia. Use the mnemonic *JAMCO* to assess for delirium or dementia:

- **J**udgment—Does the patient have insight into own behavior? Is the patient aware of danger or safety issues?
- **A**ffect—Is affect blunt, flat, inappropriate, suddenly changed, or variable?
- **M**emory—Is memory intact? Does the patient have remote memory, but not recent or immediate? Is memory better during the day?
- **C**ognition—Is the patient able to process abstract thoughts? Are thoughts fragmented or disorganized? Does the patient make up answers to questions (confabulate) to hide deficits?
- **O**rientation—Is the patient oriented to person, place, and time? Does the patient recognize family and friends?

GLASGOW COMA SCALE

The Glasgow Coma Scale is used to assess the condition of patients who have a decreased level of consciousness or who are at risk for a decreasing level of consciousness or neurologic injury. Assess each category of response, and add up the score.

Category of Response	Stimulus	Response	Score*
Eye opening	Approach to bedside	Spontaneous response	4
	Verbal command	Opening of eyes to name or command	3
	Pain	Opening of eyes only to pain	2
		Lack of eye opening to any stimulus	1
Best verbal response	Verbal questioning with maximum arousal	Appropriate orientation; conversant; correct identification of self, year, month, and place	5
		Confusion, disorientation in one or more areas, but is conversant	4

GLASGOW COMA SCALE (cont'd)

Category of Response	Stimulus	Response	Score*
		Inappropriate use of words, cursing, lack of sustained conversation	3
		Incomprehensible words, moaning	2
		Lack of sound with any stimuli	1
Best motor response	Verbal command[†] Pain (pressure on proximal nail bed)	Obedience to the command	6
		Lack of obedience but attempts to remove offending stimulus	5
		Flexion withdrawal[†]	4
		Abnormal flexion, flexing of arm at elbow and pronation, making a fist	3
		Abnormal extension, extension of arm at elbow with adduction and internal rotation of arm at shoulder	2
		Lack of response	1

*The highest possible score is 15. The higher the score, the better the condition of the patient.
[†]For example, "Raise your arm, hold up two fingers."
Adapted from Lewis SM, Dirksen SR, Heitkemper MM, et al: *Medical-surgical nursing: assessment and management of clinical problems,* ed 9, St Louis, 2014, Mosby.

"FOUR" SCORE NEUROLOGICAL ASSESSMENT SCALE

Eye Response (E)

E4	Eyelids open or opened, tracking, or blinking to command
E3	Eyelids open but not tracking
E2	Eyelids closed, open to loud voice, not tracking
E1	Eyelids closed, open to pain, not tracking
E0	Eyelids remain closed with pain

Motor Response (M)

M4	Thumbs up, fist, or peace sign to command
M3	Localizing to pain
M2	Flexion response to pain
M1	Exterior posturing
M0	No response to pain or generalized myoclonus status epilepticus

Brain Stem Reflexes (B)

B4	Pupil and corneal reflexes present
B3	One pupil wide and fixed
B2	Pupil *or* corneal reflexes absent
B1	Pupil *and* corneal reflexes absent
B0	Pupil, corneal, and cough reflexes absent

Respiration (R)

R4	Not intubated, regular breathing pattern
R3	Not intubated, Cheyne-Stokes breathing pattern
R2	Not intubated, irregular breathing pattern
R1	Breathes above ventilator rate
R0	Breathes at ventilator rate or has apnea

From Wijdicks EF, Mamlet WR, et al: Validation of new coma scale: the FOUR Score, *Ann Neurology* 58(4):585, 2005; and Wolf CA, Wijdick EF, et al: Further validation of the FOUR Score coma scale by intensive care nurses, *Mayo Clinical Procedures* 82(4):435, 2007. Reproduced by permission of Mayo Foundation for Medical Education and Research. All rights reserved.

Fall Risk Factors

The risk of falling becomes greater when a patient becomes ill. Fever, electrolyte imbalance, and dulled mental alertness often contribute to a fall, especially for the elderly patient. General factors that contribute to falls include the following:

- Medications that cause postural hypotension or dizziness; polypharmacy (sedatives, hypnotics, antihypertensives, diuretics, antidepressants, laxatives)
- Muscle weakness from inactivity or illness (stroke)
- Gait alteration due to disease or injury; neuropathy in the feet and legs (diabetes)
- Vision problems or dirty eyeglasses
- Balance or gait problem (after stroke or neurologic disorder)
- Alcohol use
- Mental changes: dementia, delirium
- Incontinence and urgency
- Neurologic diseases (stroke, Parkinson disease, multiple sclerosis, etc.)
- Illness and fever
- Severe osteoporosis and spontaneous fracture
- Environmental hazards (e.g., scatter rugs, pets, stairs, slippery floors or showers, small objects on floors, cords in pathways)
- Often, a combination of factors causes a person to fall (Figure 5-1).

Fall Risk Assessment Scale

Nursing fall risk assessment, diagnoses, and interventions are based on use of the Morse Fall Scale (MFS) (Morse, 1997; available at: http://cf.networkofcare.org/library/Morse%20Fall%20Scale.pdf). The MFS is used widely in acute care settings, both in hospital and long-term care inpatient settings. The MFS requires systematic, reliable assessment of a patient's fall risk factors upon admission, fall, change in status, and discharge or transfer to a new setting. MFS subscales include assessment of:

1. History of falling; immediate or within 3 months

No = 0
Yes = 25

2. Secondary diagnosis

No = 0
Yes = 15

3. Ambulatory aid

None, bed rest, wheelchair, nurse = 0
Crutches, cane, walker = 15
Furniture = 30

4. IV/heparin lock

No = 0
Yes = 20

5. Gait/transferring

Normal, bed rest, immobile = 0
Weak = 10
Impaired = 20

6. Mental status

Oriented to own ability = 0
Forgets limitations = 15

Risk Level	MFS Score	Action
No risk	0-24	None
Low risk	25-50	Use Standard Fall Prevention Interventions
High risk	≥51	Use High Risk Fall Prevention Interventions

Retrieved from U.S. Department of Veterans Affairs: VHA NCPS Fall Prevention and Management. http://www.patientsafety.va.gov/professionals/onthejob/falls.asp.

Fall Risk Assessment

Place a check mark in front of the items that apply to the patient.

General Information

___ Age over 70

___ History of falls*

___ Confusion at times

___ Confused most of the time*

___ Impaired memory or judgment

___ Unable to follow directions*

___ Needs assistance with elimination

___ Visual impairment

___ Feels physically weak*

Medications

___ Receiving central nervous system suppressants (narcotic, sedative, tranquilizer, hypnotic, antidepressant, psychotropic, anticonvulsant)

___ Receiving medication that causes orthostatic hypotension (antihypertensive, diuretic)*

___ Medication that may cause diarrhea (cathartic)

___ Medication that may alter blood glucose levels (insulin, hypoglycemics)

Gait and Balance

___ Poor balance when standing*

___ Balance problems when walking*

___ Swaying, lurching, or slapping gait*

___ Unstable when making turns*

___ Needs assistive device (walker, cane, holds on to furniture)*

Note: A check mark on any starred item indicates a risk for falls. A combination of four or more of the unstarred items indicates a risk for falls.

FIGURE 5-1 Fall risk assessment. (From deWit S, O'Neill P: *Fundamental concepts and skills for nursing,* ed 4, Philadelphia, 2014, Saunders.)

Pitting Edema Scale

To assess for pitting edema, depress the skin with your fingertips over the tibia or the medial malleolus for 5 seconds, and then release. Normally there is no edema except during pregnancy or when the person has been standing all day. Check all dependent areas for edema, including the sacrum.

1 + = Trace   Pit is barely seen, 2 mm depth

2 + = Mild   Pit is deeper and rebounds within a
                     few seconds, 4 mm depth

3 + = Moderate   Deep pit is formed, 6 mm depth

4 + = Severe   Deeper pit is formed that may take
                     more than 30 seconds to rebound,
                     8 mm depth

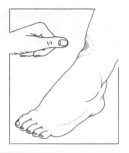

(Adapted from Christensen BL, Kockrow EO: *Foundations of nursing*, ed 6, St Louis, 2011, Mosby.)

Skin Pressure Points

Pressure points (Figure 5-2) should be examined whenever a patient is repositioned but must be assessed every 2 hours for the immobilized patient.

RISK FACTORS FOR PRESSURE ULCERS

Consider patients with the following problems as having high risk for skin breakdown and pressure ulcers:

- Immobility (e.g., stroke, paraplegia, quadriplegia, severe trauma, traction)
- Malnutrition and low body weight; hypoalbuminemia
- Dehydration
- Incontinence
- Anemia
- Peripheral vascular disease
- Diabetes mellitus
- Dementia
- Edema
- Dry skin
- Fracture
- Malignancy
- Infection

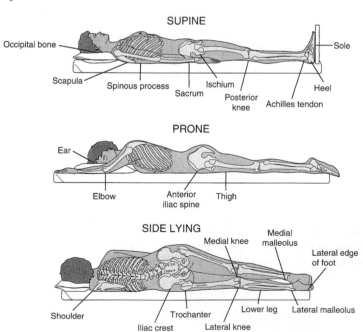

FIGURE 5-2 Pressure points.

STAGING PRESSURE ULCERS

The following staging criteria are recommended by the National Pressure Ulcer Advisory Panel and the Agency for Healthcare Research and Quality (AHRQ). Pressure ulcers, once originally staged, should not be *reverse staged*—that is, a stage IV ulcer remains a stage IV until it becomes a *healed stage IV.* Healing is documented by improvement in wound size, depth, amount of necrotic tissue, and amount of exudate. Eschar must be debrided before proper staging can occur.

Suspected deep tissue injury	Localized discolored intact skin that is maroon or purple or a blood-filled blister resulting from damage to underlying soft tissue from pressure or shear. The area may be painful, firm, mushy, boggy, warmer, or cooler when compared with adjacent tissue.
Stage I	An area of red, deep pink, or mottled skin that does not blanch with fingertip pressure. In people with darker skin, discoloration of the skin, warmth, edema, or induration may be signs of a stage I pressure ulcer.
Stage II	Partial-thickness skin loss involving epidermis, dermis, or both. May appear as an abrasion, a blister, or a shallow crater. Area around damaged skin may feel warmer.
Stage III	Full-thickness skin loss that looks like a deep crater and may extend to the fascia. Subcutaneous tissue is damaged or necrotic. Bacterial infection of the ulcer is common and causes drainage from the ulcer. There may be damage to the surrounding tissue.
Stage IV	Full-thickness skin loss with extensive tissue necrosis, or damage to muscle, bone, or supporting structures (e.g., tendon, joint capsule). Undermining and sinus tracts (tunnels) may also be present. Infection is usually widespread. The ulcer may appear dry and black, with a buildup of tough, necrotic tissue (eschar), or it can appear wet and oozing (Figure 5-3).
Unstageable	Loss of full thickness of tissue. The base of the ulcer is covered by eschar (tan, brown, or black) in the wound bed, or the base of the ulcer contains slough (yellow, tan, gray, green, or brown).

Adapted from deWit SC, O'Neill P: *Fundamental concepts and skills for nursing*, ed 4, Philadelphia, 2014, Saunders.

Substance Abuse Screening—CAGE*

Cut down: "Have you ever thought you should **cut down** on your drinking or drug use?"

Annoyed: "Have people **annoyed** you by criticizing your drinking or drug use?"

Guilty: "Have you felt bad or **guilty** about your drinking or drug use?"

Eye-opener: "Have you ever had a drink or used drugs first thing in the morning to steady your nerves or to get rid of a hangover **(eye-opener)**?"

Answering yes to any of these questions indicates that the patient may have a substance abuse problem.

*Adapted from *Mosby's PDQ for LPN*, ed 3, St Louis, 2013, Mosby.

Braden Scale

FOR PREDICTING PRESSURE SORE RISK

Patient's Name _____   Evaluator's Name _____   Date of Assessment

SENSORY PERCEPTION ability to respond meaningfully to pressure-related discomfort	1. Completely Limited: Unresponsive (does not moan, flinch, or grasp) to painful stimuli, due to diminished level of consciousness or sedation OR limited ability to feel pain over most of body surface.	2. Very Limited: Responds only to painful stimuli. Cannot communicate discomfort except by moaning or restlessness OR has a sensory impairment which limits the ability to feel pain or discomfort over 1/2 of body.	3. Slightly Limited: Responds to verbal commands, but cannot always communicate discomfort or need to be turned OR has some sensory impairment which limits ability to feel pain or discomfort in 1 or 2 extremities.	4. No Impairment: Responds to verbal commands. Has no sensory deficit which would limit ability to feel or voice pain or discomfort.				
MOISTURE degree to which skin is exposed to moisture	1. Constantly Moist: Skin is kept moist almost constantly by perspiration, urine, etc. Dampness is detected every time patient is moved or turned.	2. Very Moist: Skin is often, but not always moist. Linen must be changed at least once a shift.	3. Occasionally Moist: Skin is occasionally moist, requiring an extra linen change approximately once a day.	4. Rarely Moist: Skin is usually dry; linen only requires changing at routine intervals.				
ACTIVITY degree of physical activity	1. Bedfast: Confined to bed	2. Chairfast: Ability to walk severely limited or non-existent. Cannot bear own weight and/or must be assisted into chair or wheelchair.	3. Walks Occasionally: Walks occasionally during day, but for very short distances, with or without assistance. Spends majority of each shift in bed or chair.	4. Walks Frequently: Walks outside the room at least twice a day and inside room at least once every 2 hours during waking hours.				
MOBILITY ability to change and control body position	1. Completely Immobile: Does not make even slight changes in body or extremity position without assistance.	2. Very Limited: Makes occasional slight changes in body or extremity position but unable to make frequent or significant changes independently.	3. Slightly Limited: Makes frequent though slight changes in body or extremity position independently.	4. No Limitations: Makes major and frequent changes in position without assistance.				
NUTRITION usual food intake pattern	1. Very Poor: Never eats a complete meal. Rarely eats more than 1/3 of any food offered. Eats 2 servings or less of protein (meat or dairy products) per day. Takes fluids poorly. Does not take a liquid dietary supplement OR is NPO and/or maintained on clear liquids or IV's for more than 5 days.	2. Probably Inadequate: Rarely eats a complete meal and generally eats only about 1/2 of any food offered. Protein intake includes only 3 servings of meat or dairy products per day. Occasionally will take a dietary supplement OR receives less than optimum amount of liquid diet or tube feeding.	3. Adequate: Eats over half of most meals. Eats a total of 4 servings of protein (meat, dairy products) each day. Occasionally will refuse a meal, but will usually take a supplement if offered OR is on a tube feeding or TPN regimen that probably meets most of nutritional needs.	4. Excellent: Eats most of every meal. Never refuses a meal. Usually eats a total of 4 or more servings of meat and dairy products. Occasionally eats between meals. Does not require supplementation.				
FRICTION AND SHEAR	1. Problem: Requires moderate to maximum assistance in moving. Complete lifting without sliding against sheets is impossible. Frequently slides down in bed or chair, requiring frequent repositioning with maximum assistance. Spasticity, contractures or agitation leads to almost constant friction.	2. Potential Problem: Moves feebly or requires minimum assistance. During a move, skin probably slides to some extent against sheets, chair, restraints, or other devices. Maintains relatively good position in chair or bed most of the time but occasionally slides down.	3. No Apparent Problem: Moves in bed and in chair independently and has sufficient muscle strength to lift up completely during move. Maintains good position in bed or chair at all times.					

Total Score _____

Key: At risk, 15-18; Moderate risk, 13-14; High risk, 10-12; Severe risk, 9.

FIGURE 5-3 Braden Scale for Predicting Pressure Sore Risk. (Copyright 1988, Barbara Braden and Nancy Bergstrom. Reprinted with permission.)

Erikson's Stages of Development

Nursing students are often asked to place the patient within one of Erikson's stages of development by listing some behaviors to verify the correct stage. The following chart provides a listing of sample behaviors that are appropriate for each stage:

Verbal Behaviors	Nonverbal Behaviors
Trust vs. Mistrust (Birth to 18 Months)	
Trust	
"I believe you." "I know I can tell you…" "You will help me." "You are my friend."	Asking for help with the expectation of receiving it. Accepting help from others comfortably. Sharing time, opinions, emotions, and experiences.
Mistrust	
"I am afraid of you." "I can't tell you about anything." "You cheat."	Inability to accept help. Confining conversation to superficialities. Rigidly controlling behavior so that only that which is socially approved is exhibited. Refusal to share time, experiences, opinions, and emotions.
Autonomy vs. Shame and Doubt (1½ to 3 Years)	
Autonomy	
"I will." "I won't." "Okay, I'll do it myself." "This is my opinion." "I can wait."	Tries to dress self or perform other tasks on own. Accepting group rules but able to express dissent when it is felt. Accepting leadership role when it is appropriate. Expressing own opinion. Accepting postponement of wish gratification easily. Ability to cooperate. Demonstrates some self-control.
Shame and Doubt	
"My opinion doesn't count." "I never know the answers." "I don't want to hear what you have to say." "I must be right." "I should do that."	Overly concerned with being clean. Not maintaining own opinion when opposed. Failing to express needs. Maintaining own opinion despite adequate proof to the contrary. Lacks self-control. Unable to wait; hoarding; soiling. Being vindictive.
Initiative vs. Guilt (3 to 6 Years)	
Initiative	
"Let me try." "What is it? How does it work?" "Where does that road go?" "May I wash my hair?"	Exploring. Starting new projects with eagerness. Expressing curiosity. Being original. Ability to evaluate own behavior. Brushes teeth without being told.
Guilt	
"I'm afraid to do that." "You go first, and I will follow." "I'm ashamed to make a mistake."	Imitating others rather than developing ideas independently. Expressing a great deal of embarrassment over a small mistake. Always taking the blame.

Continued

Clinical Quick Reference

Erikson's Stages of Development (cont'd)

Verbal Behaviors	Nonverbal Behaviors

Industry vs. Inferiority (7 to 10 Years)

Industry

"I'm working on this. When it is done, I will start on that."
"I like to be busy."
"Group projects are fun."
"I'm going to do my homework now."

Completing a task once it is started. Working well with others. Using time effectively. Feelings of competence. Good self-esteem.

Inferiority

"I can't work with other people."
"I have a lot of things going but nothing finished."
"I don't think I can do it."

Not completing any set tasks. Not contributing to the work of the group. Not organizing work. Avoids responsibility.

Identity vs. Role Diffusion (10 to 17 Years)

Identity

"I'm going to be a nurse."
"I believe in these principles."
"I think mothers should do this, and fathers should do that."
"I know where I'm going."
"I feel good about myself."

Establishing relationships with the same sex and then with the opposite sex. Planning realistically for the future. Reexamining values. Asserting independence. Trying various things.

Role Diffusion

"I don't know who I am."
"Where am I going?"
"Is it better to be male or female?"
"I don't know what I mean."

Failing to differentiate roles or goals in life. Failing to assume responsibility for directing own behavior. Imitating others indiscriminately. Accepting the values of others without question.

Intimacy vs. Isolation (18 to 40 Years)

Intimacy

"We are very close friends."
"I love Dan."
"My family is very close."
"I have lots of good friends."

Establishing a close and intense relationship with another person. Acting out and accepting appropriate sexual behavior as desirable. Maintaining a marital or other monogamous relationship.

Isolation

"I'm a loner."
"I don't need anyone."
"I don't care about anyone."
"I'm very lonely."

Remaining alone. Not seeking out others for companionship or help. Avoiding sex role by remaining nondescript in mannerisms and dress.

Generativity vs. Stagnation (40 to 65 Years)

Generativity

"John and I have agreed to have two children."
"He has his work and I have mine… together we make a team."
"I am raising three children."
"I am employed at…"
"I love to sew."

Productive. Maintaining employment. Parenting. Accepting interdependence. Guiding others. Creative. Community or church leadership. Completes creative endeavors; has hobbies. Performs own self-care and takes responsibility for own health.

Erikson's Stages of Development (cont'd)

Verbal Behaviors	Nonverbal Behaviors

Stagnation

"I can't hold a job." "I don't want to learn about it." "I haven't time to volunteer." "You do it; I'm going out." "That's too bad, but it isn't my problem."	Not listening to others because of need to talk about oneself. Constantly losing employment. Showing concern only for oneself despite the needs of others. Self-absorption. Always finds excuses. Refuses to learn self-care.

Integrity vs. Despair (65 Years to Death)

Integrity

"Life has been very good to me." "I can't do the things I once did, but I enjoy other things." "I enjoy discussing current events." "I read the newspaper every day." "I love watching the birds at the feeder." "I enjoy seeing my children and my grandchildren."	Using past experiences to guide others. Accepting new ideas. Accepting limitations. Maintaining productivity in some area. Exploring philosophy of living and dying. Enjoying some aspect of things as they are. Actively participating in own care as much as able.

Despair

"I am no use to anyone." "Everyone is gone...my family, my friends." "What is the use of living; I can't do anything." "Everything I did is gone now. Why did this happen?" "These new ways are no good."	Crying; being apathetic and listless. Not developing any new interests beyond a few routine activities. Developing no new relationships. Not accepting changes. Limiting interpersonal contacts. Demanding unnecessary help and attention. Remaining in pajamas and robe all the time.

Piaget's Cognitive Developmental Stages

Stage	Characterized By
Sensorimotor Birth to 2 years	Begins to differentiate self from others and objects. Recognizes self as agent of action and starts acting intentionally with simple repetitive actions; shakes a rattle to make noise. Object permanence is achieved; understands that things still exist even when no longer within range of vision. Egocentric.
Preoperational 2 to 7 years	Learns to use language; represents objects with images and words (uses symbols while thinking). Still egocentric in thinking; has difficulty in taking the viewpoint of others. Thinks others see the world as he/she does.
Concrete operational 7 to 11 years	Reasoning and thought become logical, but limited to own experience. Understands cause and effect. Can classify objects according to several features and has ability to order them in series such as by size. By age 6 achieves conservation of number; by age 7, conservation of mass; and by age 9, conservation of weight.

Continued

Piaget's Cognitive Developmental Stages (cont'd)

Stage	Characterized By
Formal operational 11 years and up	Acquires ability to develop abstract concepts for self. Oriented to problem solving. Grows to be concerned with the hypothetical, the future, and 　　ideological matters.

Data from Leifer G: *Introduction to maternity & pediatric nursing,* ed 7, St Louis, 2015, Mosby; Potter PA, et al: *Basic nursing,* ed 7, St Louis, 2012, Mosby; Atherton JS: *Learning and teaching: Piaget's developmental theory.* http://www.learningandteaching.info/learning/piaget.htm, 2011.

Child Abuse and Neglect

One sign by itself does not necessarily indicate a problem, but be alert for the following signs, which call for a more in-depth assessment for possible abuse:

- Suspicious bruises, lacerations, burns, fractures, or head injury
- Welts, bite marks, or clumps of hair loss
- Abdominal injury with suspicious history
- Repeated or multiple fractures without an adequate history of precipitating events
- Unkempt or dirty appearance, inappropriate clothing for the weather
- Failure to thrive
- Wariness or clinging to adults who are strangers or getting upset when another child cries
- Fearfulness of parents or other adults
- A sophisticated knowledge of sexual activities
- Promiscuity and defiance of authority
- Adult behavior such as belittling the child, constantly blaming the child, repeatedly embarrassing the child, or withholding love and affection from the child

Remember that some odd skin markings can be from a cultural practice such as "coining," in which a coin is rubbed over the skin to help relieve illness. This practice is not abuse. If signs of abuse are definite, they must be reported.

Elder Abuse and Neglect

One sign alone does not necessarily indicate abuse, but some telltale signs that there could be a problem are as follows:

- Bruises, black eyes, lacerations, puncture wounds, pressure marks, broken bones, burns, abrasions
- Signs of marks from restraints
- Untreated injuries in various stages of healing
- Sprains, dislocations, or internal injuries
- Pressure ulcers, poor hygiene, or unattended medical needs
- Bruises around the genital area or breasts
- Unusual weight loss in combination with other signs
- Unkempt; inappropriate dress or hygiene
- Unusual fear exhibited
- An unexplained extreme withdrawal from usual activities

- Abrupt change in behavior
- A sudden change in alertness and indications of depression (may indicate emotional abuse)
- Inappropriate clothing for the weather
- Dehydration and/or malnutrition
- Broken eyeglasses
- Medication overdose or underutilization
- Caregiver refusal to allow visitors to see elderly person alone
- Sudden changes in financial situation
- Caregiver or spouse behavior such as belittling or threats
- Strained or tense relationships, frequent arguments with the caregiver or spouse

■ PAIN

The Joint Commission (TJC) Pain Standards

The following is a summary of the standards for pain assessment for all patients in any setting from TJC:

1. Patients have the right to appropriate assessment and management of pain.
2. Pain will be assessed in all patients in a timely and recurring manner.
3. Policies and procedures must support safe medication prescription or ordering.
4. Patients must be educated, as appropriate, about pain and managing pain as part of treatment.
5. The discharge process will provide for continuing pain care based on the patient's assessed needs at the time of discharge.
6. Organizations will collect data to monitor their performance, addressing the following areas:
   - Appropriate pain assessment and management
   - Effective pain treatment or referral for treatment
   - Timely assessment and reassessment of pain, including the nature and intensity
   - Patient involvement in making decisions about pain management
   - Education for staff and patients regarding the following:
     - The importance of effective pain management
     - Pain management as a part of total treatment
     - Continuing pain care after discharge
     - Documentation of pain assessments, treatments, and evaluation of effectiveness
     - Staff competency in pain assessment and management

Pain is considered the fifth vital sign and should be assessed whenever vital signs are taken. After assessment, documentation of the findings must be completed. Numerous pain assessment tools are available. Use the scale that is designated in the pain assessment procedure for your agency.

Focused Assessment for the Patient with Pain*

LOCATION
- Where is your pain?
- Does the pain radiate (e.g., into arms, back, down legs, etc.)?

CHARACTERISTICS
- Describe your pain.
- What words would describe your pain (e.g., aching, burning, gnawing, sharp, dull, continuous, intermittent)?

QUANTITY
- Use a pain scale (e.g., numeric, descriptive).

PATTERN
- When did the pain start?
- Did the pain begin during or after an activity or eating?
- Did the pain start suddenly?
- Has the pain increased over time?

ASSOCIATED FACTORS
- Have you had other symptoms (e.g., shortness of breath, nausea, vomiting, palpitations, or sweating)?

ALLEVIATING FACTORS
- What have you used to relieve the pain (e.g., over-the-counter [OTC] medications, position change)?
- Did the measures that you tried provide relief?

AGGRAVATING FACTORS
- What (if anything) makes the pain worse?

---

*Modified from deWit SC: *Medical-surgical nursing: concepts and practice*, ed 2, St Louis, 2013, Saunders.

Pain Rating Scales

NUMERIC PAIN SCALE
The patient rates the pain on a scale of 1 to 10, with 1 being almost no pain and 10 being unbearable pain.

UNIVERSAL PAIN ASSESSMENT

UNIVERSAL PAIN ASSESSMENT TOOL

This pain assessment tool is intended to help patient care providers assess pain according to individual patient needs. Explain and use 0–10 Scale for patient self-assessment. Use the faces or behavioral observations to interpret expressed pain when patient cannot communicate his/her pain intensity.

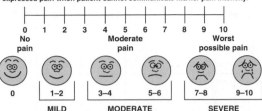

		MILD		MODERATE		SEVERE	
ACTIVITY TOLERANCE SCALE	NO PAIN	CAN BE IGNORED	INTERFERES WITH TASKS	INTERFERES WITH CONCENTRATION	INTERFERES WITH BASIC NEEDS	BEDREST REQUIRED	
SPANISH	NADA DE DOLOR	UN POQUITO DE DOLOR	UN DOLOR LEVE	DOLOR FUERTE	DOLOR DEMASIADO FUERTE	UN DOLOR INSOPORTABLE	
FRENCH	AUCUNE DOULEUR	LÉGÈRE DOULEUR	DOULEUR MODÉRÉE	FORTE DOULEUR	TRÈS FORTE DOULEUR	DOULEUR EXTREME	
GERMAN	KEINE SCHMERZEN	LEICHTE SCHMERZEN	MÄSSIGE SCHMERZEN	STARKE SCHMERZEN	SEHR STARKE SCHMERZEN	EXTREME SCHMERZEN	
JAPANESE	痛みなし	軽い痛み	中程度の痛み	ひどい痛み	非常にひどい痛み	最悪の痛み	
TAGALOG	HINDI MASAKIT	KAUNTIG SAKIT	MEDYO MASAKIT	TALAGANG MASAKIT	MASAKITNA MASAKIT	PINAKAMASAKIT	
HINDI	DARDNAHI HAI	BAHUT KAM	HILNE SE TAKLEF HOTI HAI	SOCH NAHIN SAKTE	KUCH NAHIN KAR SAKTE	DARD BAHUT HAI	

(Reprinted with permission from UCLA Department of Anesthesiology, David Geffen School of Medicine at UCLA: The Wong-Baker FACES Rating Scale; adapted from Hockenberry MJ, Wilson D: *Wong's nursing care of infants and children,* ed 9, St Louis, 2011, Mosby.)

DESCRIPTIVE WORD RATING SCALE

Chart rating over scale (e.g., 3/5).

0	1	2	3	4	5
No pain	Mild	Discomforting	Distressing	Horrible	Excruciating

VISUAL ANALOG SCALE (VAS)

Have the patient indicate the degree of pain by marking the line below:

No pain at all_____Greatest pain possible

VERBAL DESCRIPTOR SCALE (VDS)

Have the patient check the best descriptor of his or her pain at this moment (may read to the resident):

____ absent
____ minimal
____ mild
____ moderate
____ fairly severe

____ severe
____ very severe
____ extremely severe
____ exquisite
____ unbearable

Clinical Quick Reference

NEONATAL/INFANT PAIN SCALE (NIPS)

Pain Assessment Tools
Neonatal/Infant Pain Scale (NIPS)
(Recommended for children less than 1 year old)—A score greater than 3 indicates pain

Pain Assessment		Score
Facial Expression		
0 – Relaxed muscles	Restful face, neutral expression	
1 – Grimace	Tight facial muscles; furrowed brow, chin, jaw (negative facial expression—nose, mouth and brow)	
Cry		
0 – No Cry	Quiet, not crying	
1 – Whimper	Mild moaning, intermittent	
2 – Vigorous Cry	Loud scream; rising, shrill, continuous (Note: Silent cry may be scored if baby is intubated as evidenced by obvious mouth and facial movement)	
Breathing Patterns		
0 – Relaxed	Usual pattern for this infant	
1 – Change in Breathing	Indrawing, irregular, faster than usual; gagging; breath holding	
Arms		
0 – Relaxed/Restrained	No muscular rigidity; occasional random movements of arms	
1 – Flexed/Extended	Tense, straight legs; rigid and/or rapid extension, flexion	
Legs		
0 – Relaxed/Restrained	No muscular rigidity; occasional random leg movement	
1 – Flexed/Extended	Tense, straight legs; rigid and/or rapid extension, flexion	
State of Arousal		
0 – Sleeping/Awake	Quiet, peaceful, sleeping or alert, random leg movement	
1 – Fussy	Alert, restless, and thrashing	

(From Lawrence J, Alcock D, McGrath P, et al: The development of a tool to assess neonatal pain, 1993, *Neonatal Network* 12(6):59-66. Reprinted with permission from Children's Hospital of Eastern Ontario, Ottawa, Ontario, Canada.)

REVISED FLACC SCALE

	0	1	2
F—Face	No particular expression or smile	Occasional grimace or frown, withdrawn, disinterested *Appears sad or worried*	Frequent-to-constant frown, clenched jaw, quivering chin *Distress-looking face: expression of fright or panic*
L—Legs	Normal position or relaxed	Uneasy, restless, tense *Occasional tremors*	Kicking or legs drawn up *Marked increase in spasticity, constant tremors or jerking*
A—Activity	Lying quietly, normal position, moves easily	Squirming, shifting back and forth, tense *Mildly agitated (e.g., head back and forth, aggression); shallow, splinting respirations; intermittent sighs*	Arched, rigid, or jerking *Severe agitation, head banging, shivering (not rigors); breath-holding, gasping or sharp intake of breath; severe splinting*
C—Cry	No crying (awake or asleep)	Moans or whimpers, occasional complaint *Occasional verbal outburst or grunt*	Crying steadily, screams or sobs, frequent complaints *Repeated outbursts, constant grunting*
C—Consolability	Content, relaxed	Reassured by occasional touching, hugging, or talking to; distractible	Difficult to console or comfort *Pushing away caregiver, resisting care or comfort measures*

Each of the five categories is scored from 0-2, which results in a total score between 0 and 10.

Patients who are awake: Observe for at least 1-2 minutes. Observe legs and body uncovered. Reposition patient or observe activity, assess body for tenseness and tone. Initiate consoling interventions if needed.

Patients who are asleep: Observe for at least 2 minutes or longer. Observe body and legs uncovered. If possible reposition the patient. Touch the body and assess for tenseness and tone.

The revised FLACC can be used for all nonverbal children. The additional descriptors (in bold) are descriptors validated in children with cognitive impairment. The nurse can review with parents the descriptors within each category. Ask them if there are additional behaviors that are better indicators of pain in their child. Add these behaviors to the tool in the appropriate category.

Clinical Quick Reference

FLACC BEHAVIORAL PAIN SCALE

F—FACE

Score 0 points if patient has a relaxed face, eye contact, and interest in surroundings

Score 1 point if patient has a worried look to face, with eyebrows lowered, eyes partially closed, cheeks raised, mouth pursed

Score 2 points if patient has deep furrows in the forehead, with closed eyes, open mouth, and deep lines around nose/lips

L—LEGS

Score 0 points if patient has usual tone and motion to limbs (legs and arms)

Score 1 point if patient has increase tone, rigidity, tense, intermittent flexion/extension of limbs

Score 2 points if patient has hypertonicity, legs pulled tight, exaggerated flexion/extension of limbs, tremors

A—ACTIVITY

Score 0 points if patient moves easily and freely, normal activity/restrictions

Score 1 point if patient shifts positions, hesitant to move, guarding, tense torso, pressure on body part

Score 2 points if patient is in fixed position, rocking, side-to-side head movement, rubbing body part

C—CRY

Score 0 points if patient has no cry/moan awake or asleep

Score 1 point if patient has occasional moans, cries, whimpers, sighs

Score 2 points if patient has frequent/continuous moans, cries, grunts

C—CONSOLABILITY

Score 0 points if patient is calm and does not require consoling

Score 1 point if patient responds to comfort by touch or talk in $\frac{1}{2}$-1 minute

Score 2 points if patient require constant consoling or is unconsoled after an extended time

Whenever feasible, behavioral measurement of pain should be used in conjunction with self-report. When self-report is not possible, interpretation of pain behaviors and decision making regarding treatment of pain requires careful consideration of the context in which the pain behaviors were observed.

Each category is scored on the 0-2 scale, which results in a total score of 0-10.

ASSESSMENT OF BEHAVIORAL SCORE

0 = Relaxed and comfortable

1-3 = Mild discomfort

4-6 = Moderate pain

7-10 = Severe discomfort/pain

MEMORY DEVICE FOR ASSESSMENT OF PAIN: PQRST

Factor	Questions to Ask
P—Precipitating events	What events or factors (e.g., activity, exercise, resting) precipitated the pain or discomfort?
Q—Quality of pain or discomfort	What does the pain or discomfort feel like (e.g., dull, aching, sharp, tight)?
R—Radiation of pain	Where is the pain located? Where does the pain radiate to (e.g., back, arms, jaw, teeth, shoulder, elbow)?
S—Severity of pain	On a scale of 0 to 10 with 10 being the most severe pain, how would you rate the pain or discomfort?
T—Timing	When did the pain or discomfort begin? Has the pain changed since that time? Have you had pain like this before?

This memory device may be used for pain in other locations as well.
Adapted from Lewis SM, et al: *Medical-surgical nursing: assessment and management of clinical problems,* ed 9, St Louis, 2014, Mosby.

MEASURES TO RELIEVE PAIN AND DISCOMFORT

- Relieve extraneous sensory input by providing a quiet, tidy environment.
- Administer pain medication promptly; reassess patient for pain level in 30 minutes (depending on route) and at the time the next dose should be given.
- Advise patient to ask for pain medication before pain becomes severe; medication is more effective if given before the onset of severe pain.
- Provide distraction with reading material, a TV program, pleasant music, a game, or conversation.
- Offer a massage.
- Teach relaxation exercises.
- Assist with a pleasant imagery exercise.
- Straighten bed linens and position for comfort.
- Seek to reduce anxieties if possible.
- Encourage verbalization of fears.
- Provide other analgesics between narcotic doses, if ordered.
- Encourage use of heat or cold treatments as ordered.
- Determine whether pain medication ordered is effective; if not, request an order change from the physician.
- Remember that just because a patient may go to sleep, it does not mean that the pain medication is not needed.

MNEMONIC FOR CHARTING PAIN ASSESSMENT: OLDCART

- **O**nset
- **L**ocation
- **D**uration
- **C**haracteristics
- **A**ggravating factors
- **R**elieving factors
- **T**reatments

Equianalgesic Doses of Opioids

Drug and Route*	Equianalgesic Dose (mg)[†]	TIME COURSE OF ANALGESIC EFFECTS		
		Onset (min)	Peak (min)	Duration (hr)
Codeine				
PO	200	30-45	60-120	4-6
IM	130	10-30	30-60	4-6
Subcut	130	10-30	30-60	4-6
Hydrocodone				
PO	30	10-30	30-60	4-6
Hydromorphone				
PO	7.5	30	90-120	4
IM	1.5	15	30-60	4-5
IV	1.5	10-15	15-30	2-3
Subcut	1.5	15	30-90	4
Levorphanol				
PO	4	10-60	90-120	6-8
IM	2	—	60	6-8
IV	2	—	Within 20	6-8
Subcut	2	—	60-90	6-8
Methadone				
PO	20	30-60	90-120	6-8
IM	10	10-20	60-120	4-5
IV	10	—	15-30	3-4[‡]
Morphine				
PO	30	—	60-120	3-5
IM	10	10-30	30-60	3-5
IV	10	—	20	3-5
Subcut	10	10-30	50-90	3-5
Epidural	—	15-60	—	Up to 24
Intrathecal	—	15-60	—	Up to 24
Oxycodone				
PO	10	15-30	60	3-6[§]
Oxymorphone				
IM	1	10-15	30-90	4-6
IV	1	5-10	15-30	3-4
Subcut	1	10-20	—	4-6
Rectal	10	15-30	120	3-6

Use of meperidine is not recommended.

*IM administration should be avoided whenever possible.

[†]Dose in milligrams that produces a degree of analgesia equivalent to that produced by a 10-mg IM dose of morphine.

[‡]With repeated doses, methadone's duration of action may increase up to 48 hours.

[§]Effects of extended-release formulations may persist for 8 to 12 hours.

Adapted from Lehne RA: *Pharmacology for nursing care,* ed 8, Philadelphia, 2013, Saunders, and Hodgson BB, Kizior RJ: *Saunders nursing drug handbook 2014,* St Louis, 2014, Elsevier.

■ BASIC NURSING CARE

Routine Observation of Chest Tubes

- Assess respiratory status.
- Assess for pain and discomfort; medicate as needed.
- Encourage patient to cough and deep breathe.
- Patient should be in Fowler or high-Fowler position.
- Observe occlusive dressing over insertion site and surrounding skin.
- Observe tubing for kinks or obstructions; all connections should be intact and taped.
- Chest drainage collection unit should be below level of chest and upright.
- Add sterile water as needed to water-seal chamber.
- Observe the type and amount of drainage (expect less than 50 to 200 mL/hr dark red blood immediately after surgery; amount of drainage should decrease with time).
- Apply a strip of tape to the drainage unit, and mark the level of drainage for each shift.
- Observe for and expect some gentle intermittent bubbling and fluctuation in water-seal chamber unless suction is applied.
- No fluctuation suggests a blockage within system or resolution of collapsed lung.
- Continuous or rigorous bubbling suggests leakage in the system (may require retaping of connections or locating air leak using a clamp; notify RN for assistance).

Other Tips for Chest Tube Care

- Tubing is not routinely stripped or milked.
- Clamps are kept at the bedside for practitioner assessment and special procedures, but chest clamps are **not** routinely clamped.
- Drainage chamber is not routinely emptied, unless it overflows (overflow is not expected).
- If the wall suction is temporarily disconnected, the water seal remains intact; however, if the system accidentally breaks or tubing becomes disconnected, reestablish the water seal by temporarily placing the distal end of tubing in a container of sterile water.

Assisting the Patient to Urinate

With the patient positioned for urination:

- Run water in a nearby sink.
- Have a female patient blow through a straw into a glass of water.
- Assist a male patient to stand at the bedside (with a physician's order).
- Allow privacy if patient can be left alone.
- Gently, but firmly, use Credé movements over the bladder (massage from top of bladder to bottom by rocking the palm of the hand over it).
- Place patient in a warm sitz bath (with physician's order). Encourage to void into the sitz bath. Cleanse perineum afterward.
- Pour warm water over the perineum with patient attempting to void. Place the patient's hand in a bowl or pan of warm water.
- Encourage patient to breathe deep and relax; ask patient to visualize running water in a peaceful place.

Relieving Flatulence (Gas)

- Have the patient ambulate in an upright position as much as possible.
- Seek an order for simethicone medication to decrease gas formation.
- Have the patient avoid carbonated beverages, beverages containing ice, and gas-forming foods.
- Have the patient avoid drinking through a straw (it increases the swallowing of air, which causes gas).
- Use abdominal massage if not contraindicated; massage with a circular motion over the large intestine, moving in the direction that intestinal contents travel. Massage encourages gas to move down the intestinal tract.
- Use measures to stimulate a bowel movement, such as warm water with lemon juice orally, a rectal suppository (if ordered), or measures that usually work for the particular patient.
- Obtain an order for the insertion of a rectal tube.
- If discomfort is severe, ask the physician whether the patient can be placed in Trendelenburg position for short periods to encourage gas to move out of the intestine. (With the intestine and rectum higher than the stomach and head, the gas will move up and out.)

■ EMERGENCIES AND CRITICAL CARE

Nursing Actions in Case of Fire—RACE

Rescue any patients in immediate danger by removing them from the area.
Activate the fire alarm system, and notify the telephone operator.
Contain the fire by closing doors and any open windows.
Extinguish the flames with an appropriate fire extinguisher.

Calling a "Code"

If the patient does not respond to your verbal call, follow basic cardiopulmonary resuscitation (CPR) guidelines. Turn on the call light, shout (if patient is in the bathroom, activate the bathroom call bell, which does not turn off until someone turns it off), or press the code button on the room wall, or use the phone to call in a code and alert the rapid response team as you begin to do the following:

- Feel for a carotid pulse in an adult or a brachial pulse in an infant.
- Begin CPR (if patient is pulseless), and continue until relieved.
- Give chest compressions at a rate of 100 compressions per minute.
- Give ventilations at a rate of 30 compressions and then 2 ventilations.

Evaluating an ECG Rhythm Strip

When working with patients on telemetry or in the emergency department, you need to be able to do a basic evaluation of an electrocardiographic (ECG) tracing (Figure 5-4).

The following steps provide the needed data regarding the rate, rhythm, PR interval, duration of the QRS complex, and whether irregular beats are present:

- Obtain a 6-second strip (one with at least 10 large graph squares).
- Calculate the heart rate. Count the number of R waves and multiply by 10.
- Determine if rate is regular or irregular.

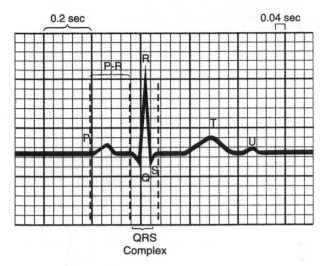

FIGURE 5-4 Normal electrocardiogram tracing.

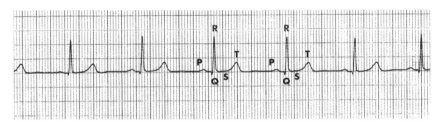

1. Rate between 50-100 bpm and regular.
2. P wave precedes each QRS complex; PR interval between 0.12-0.20 sec (3-5 small squares).
3. QRS duration between 0.04-0.12 sec (1-3 small squares).
4. QRS complexes have essentially the same shape.

FIGURE 5-5 Interpreting an electrocardiogram. (From Lewis SM, et al: *Medical-surgical nursing: assessment and management of clinical problems,* ed 9, St Louis, 2014, Mosby.)

- Is there a p wave in front of every QRS? (If not, this finding is significant.)
- Measure the PR interval. Is it normal (0.12 to 0.20 sec)? Does it vary?
- Measure the QRS duration. Is it normal (0.04 to 0.12 sec)? Measure with calipers from R wave to R wave throughout the tracing to determine whether the rate is regular. Are there premature QRS complexes? Do all the QRS complexes look the same?
- Figure 5-5 shows the results of an analysis of a normal sinus rhythm.

Telemetry Monitoring

When the patient is started on cardiac telemetry monitoring, one of two leads is most commonly used with either two electrodes or three electrodes and a ground

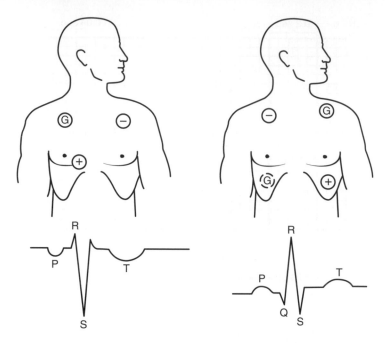

Placement of MCL₁ electrodes   Placement of lead II electrodes

FIGURE 5-6 Placement of most commonly used telemetry leads. (Adapted from Black JM, Hawks JH: *Medical-surgical nursing: clinical management for positive outcomes,* ed 7, Philadelphia, 2005, Saunders.)

being attached to the patient (Figure 5-6). **Check your hospital's procedure guide.**

Care and Observation during a Seizure

- Assist the patient to a lying position, move objects out of the way, and loosen any tight clothing.
- Do not restrain the patient.
- Place something soft under the head, if possible, such as a pillow, folded towel, or piece of clothing.
- Gently turn the head to the side to prevent aspiration of saliva.
- Do not force anything into the mouth; if the teeth are not clenched, place a soft object such as a washcloth between the teeth to protect the tongue.
- Note the times that the seizure begins and ends.
- Note the progression of movements because this is important information for the physician.
- Call for assistance, but stay with the patient.
- Remember that respirations are sometimes irregular or cease during a seizure for a short period.
- Note if the patient becomes incontinent.
- Provide privacy if possible.
- Reassure the patient that you are there.

- After the seizure is over, reorient the patient, and tell him or her that a seizure has occurred.
- Record in detail all observations of the seizure.

■ MEASUREMENTS AND CONVERSIONS

Temperature

Convert Celsius readings to Fahrenheit by multiplying the Celsius reading by 1.8 and adding 32:

$$F = (C \times 1.8) + 32$$

Convert Fahrenheit readings to Celsius by subtracting 32 from the Fahrenheit reading and dividing it by 1.8:

$$C = (F - 32)/1.8$$

Celsius (Centigrade)	Fahrenheit
36.0	96.8
36.5	97.7
37.0	98.6 (normal)
37.5	99.5
38.0	100.4
38.5	101.3
39.0	102.2
39.5	103.1
40.0	104.0
40.5	104.9
41.0	105.8
41.5	106.7
42.0	107.6

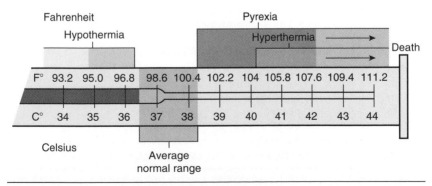

(From Perry AG, Potter PA, Elkin MK: *Nursing interventions & clinical skills,* ed 5, St Louis, 2011, Mosby.)

Time

Common Time	24-Hour Time	Common Time	24-Hour Time	Common Time	24-Hour Time
1:00 AM	0100	10:00 AM	1000	6:00 PM	1800
2:00 AM	0200	11:00 AM	1100	7:00 PM	1900
3:00 AM	0300	12:00 PM	1200	8:00 PM	2000
4:00 AM	0400	(noon)		9:00 PM	2100
5:00 AM	0500	1:00 PM	1300	10:00 PM	2200
6:00 AM	0600	2:00 PM	1400	11:00 PM	2300
7:00 AM	0700	3:00 PM	1500	12:00 AM	2400
8:00 AM	0800	4:00 PM	1600	(midnight)	
9:00 AM	0900	5:00 PM	1700		

Apothecary and Metric Equivalents

WEIGHT

METRIC		APOTHECARY*
Gram (g)	Milligram (mg)	Grain (gr)
1	1000	15
0.5	500	$7\frac{1}{2}$
0.3	300-325[†]	5
0.1	100	$1\frac{1}{2}$
0.06	60-64[†]	1
0.03	30-32[†]	$\frac{1}{2}$
0.015	15-16[†]	$\frac{1}{4}$
0.010	10	$\frac{1}{6}$
0.0006	0.6	$\frac{1}{100}$
0.0004	0.4	$\frac{1}{200}$
0.0003	0.3	$\frac{1}{200}$

*Apothecary measurements are not within recommended use but may occasionally be encountered.
[†]Measurements between systems are not always precise, therefore a range is presented.

VOLUME EQUIVALENTS: LIQUID CONVERSION

30 mL	=	1 oz (fl) = 2 tbsp (T) = 6 tsp (t)
15 mL	=	$\frac{1}{2}$ oz = 1 T = 3 t
1000 mL	=	1 quart (qt) = 1 liter (L)
500 mL	=	1 pint (pt)
5 mL	=	1 tsp (t)
4 mL	=	1 fl dr (fl D)
1 mL	=	15 (16) minims = 15 (16) drops (gtt)

From Kee J, Hayes E, McCuistion L: *Pharmacology: a nursing process approach,* ed 8, Philadelphia, 2015, Saunders.

■ COMMON LABORATORY TEST VALUES

Critical abnormal test values must be reported to the physician as soon as they are received. Check your agency's list of what tests are considered critical.

Complete Blood Count (CBC)

	Conventional Units		SI Units
Cell Counts			
Erythrocytes (RBCs)			
Male adults	$4.6\text{-}6.2$ million/mm^3		$4.6\text{-}6.2 \times 10^{12}$/L
Female adults	$4.2\text{-}5.4$ million/mm^3		$4.2\text{-}5.4 \times 10^{12}$/L
Children (varies with age)	$4.5\text{-}5.1$ million/mm^3		$4.5\text{-}5.1 \times 10^{12}$/L
Leukocytes (WBCs)			
Total	$4500\text{-}11{,}000$/mm^3		$4.5\text{-}11.0 \times 10^9$/L
Differential	Percentage	Absolute	
Myelocytes	0	0/mm^3	0/L
Band neutrophils	3-5	$150\text{-}400$/mm^3	$150\text{-}400 \times 10^6$/L
Segmented neutrophils	54-62	$3000\text{-}5800$/mm^3	$3000\text{-}5800 \times 10^6$/L
Lymphocytes	25-33	$1500\text{-}3000$/mm^3	$1500\text{-}3000 \times 10^6$/L
Monocytes	3-7	$300\text{-}500$/mm^3	$300\text{-}500 \times 10^6$/L
Eosinophils	1-3	$50\text{-}250$/mm^3	$50\text{-}250 \times 10^9$/L
Basophils	0-1	$15\text{-}50$/mm^3	$15\text{-}50 \times 10^9$/L
Platelets			
	$150{,}000\text{-}400{,}000$/mm^3		$150\text{-}350 \times 10^9$/L
Reticulocytes			
	$25{,}000\text{-}75{,}000$/mm^3 ($0.5\text{-}1.5\%$ of erythrocytes)		$25\text{-}75 \times 10^9$/L
Hemoglobin			
Male adults	$13.0\text{-}18.0$ g/dL		$8.1\text{-}11.2$ mmol/L
Female adults	$12.0\text{-}16.0$ g/dL		$7.4\text{-}9.9$ mmol/L
Newborn	$16.5\text{-}19.5$ g/dL		$10.2\text{-}12.1$ mmol/L
Children (varies with age)	$11.2\text{-}16.5$ g/dL		$7.0\text{-}10.2$ mmol/L
Fetal total	Less than 1.0% of total		Less than 0.01% of total
Hematocrit			
Male adults	$40\text{-}54$ mL/dL		$0.40\text{-}0.54$
Female adults	$37\text{-}47$ mL/dL		$0.37\text{-}0.47$
Newborn	$49\text{-}54$ mL/dL		$0.49\text{-}0.54$
Children (varies with age)	$35\text{-}49$ mL/dL		$0.35\text{-}0.49$

Corpuscular Values of Erythrocytes (for adults; values vary with age in children)

	Conventional Units	SI Units
MCH (mean corpuscular hemoglobin)	$26\text{-}34$ pg/cell	$26\text{-}34$ pg/cell
MCV (mean corpuscular volume)	$80\text{-}96$ μm^3	$80\text{-}96$ fl
MCHC (mean corpuscular hemoglobin concentration)	$32\text{-}36$ g/dL	$320\text{-}360$ g/L

Adapted from Bope ET, Kellerman RD: *Conn's current therapy 2012*, Philadelphia, 2012, Saunders.

Clinical Quick Reference

Routine Urinalysis

Component	Normal Value(s)
Color	Pale yellow to deep amber
Turbidity	Clear
Specific gravity	1.005-1.030
Osmolality	275-295 mOsm/L
pH	4.6-8.0
Glucose	Negative
Ketones	Negative
Protein	Negative
Bilirubin	Negative
Red blood cells	None to 2 per high-power field
White blood cells	None to 5 per high-power field
Bacteria	None
Casts	Few or none
Crystals	None

From Ignatavicius DD, Workman ML: *Medical-surgical nursing: patient-centered collaborative care,* ed 7, Philadelphia, 2013, Saunders.

Laboratory Values for Chemistry Panel Test (SMAC)

	Conventional Units	SI Units
Electrolytes		
Sodium, serum	135-145 mEq/L	135-145 mmol/L
Potassium, serum	3.5-5.0 mEq/L	3.5-5.0 mmol/L
Chloride, serum	96-106 mEq/L	90-106 mmol/L
Calcium, serum	8.4-10.6 mg/dL	2.10-2.65 mmol/L
Chemical Values		
Glucose, serum (fasting)	70-110 mg/dL	3.9-6.1 mmol/L
Creatinine, serum	0.6-1.2 mg/dL	50-110 µmol/L
Uric acid, serum	2.4-7.0 mg/dL	143-416 µmol/L
Blood urea nitrogen (BUN), serum	11-23 mg/dL	8.0-16.4 µmol/L
Bilirubin, total serum	0.3-1.1 mg/dL	5.1-19 mmol/L
Carbon dioxide, serum	24-31 mEq/L	24-31 mmol/L
Total protein, serum	6.0-8.0 g/dL	60-80 g/L
Albumin (A), serum	3.5-5.2 g/dL	35-52 g/L
Globulin (G), serum	2.5 g% of protein	
A/G ratio	1.5:1 to 2.5:1	
Alanine aminotransferase (ALT), serum (SGPT)	1-45 units/L	1-45 units/L
Aspartate aminotransferase (AST), serum (SGOT)	1-36 units/L	1-36 units/L
Cholesterol		
Total cholesterol, serum	<200 mg/dL	<5.20 mmol/L
Low-density lipoprotein	60-129 mg/dL	600-1290 mg/L (LDL) cholesterol, serum
High-density lipoprotein	>50-80 mg/dL	>500-800 mg/L (HDL) cholesterol, serum
Triglycerides, serum	40-150 mg/dL	0.4-1.5 g/L

SMAC, Sequential multiple analyzer computer.

Normal and Abnormal Values for Arterial Blood Gases (ABGs)*

Acid-Base Disturbances	pH	Paco$_2$ (mm Hg)	HCO$_3$ (mEq/L)	Pao$_2$	Common Causes
None (normal values)	7.35-7.45	35-45	22-26	80%-100%	
Respiratory acidosis	↓	↑	Normal		Respiratory depression (drugs, central nervous system trauma), pulmonary disease (pneumonia, chronic obstructive pulmonary disease, respiratory underventilation)
Respiratory alkalosis	↑	↓	Normal		Hyperventilation (emotions, pain, respirator overventilation)
Metabolic acidosis	↓	Normal	↓		Diabetes, shock, renal failure, intestinal fistula
Metabolic alkalosis	↑	Normal	↑		Sodium bicarbonate overdose, prolonged vomiting, nasogastric drainage

*Values may vary slightly among laboratories.
From Pagana KD, Pagana TJ: *Mosby's diagnostic and laboratory test reference,* ed 11, St Louis, 2013, Mosby.

Reference Values for Therapeutic Drug Monitoring

Therapeutic Test (Serum) for:	Range	Toxic Levels	Proprietary Test Name(s)
Antibiotic Medications			
Amikacin	20-30 mcg/mL	Peak > 35 mcg/mL* Trough > 10 mcg/mL	Amikin
Gentamicin	5-10 mcg/mL	Peak > 10 mcg/mL Trough > 2 mcg/mL	Garamycin
Tobramycin	5-10 mcg/mL	Peak > 10 mcg/mL Trough > 2 mcg/mL	Nebcin
Vancomycin	5-35 mcg/mL	Peak > 40 mcg/mL Trough > 10 mcg/mL	
Anticonvulsant Medications			
Carbamazepine	5-12 mcg/mL	>15 mcg/mL	Tegretol
Ethosuximide	40-100 mcg/mL	>250 mcg/mL	Zarontin
Phenobarbital	15-40 mcg/mL	40-100 mcg/mL (varies widely)	Luminal
Phenytoin	10-20 mcg/mL	>20 mcg/mL	Dilantin
Primidone	5-12 mcg/mL	>15 mcg/mL	Mysoline
Valproic acid	50-100 mcg/mL	>100 mcg/mL	Depakene
Analgesic Medications			
Acetaminophen	10-40 mcg/mL	>150 mcg/mL	Tylenol, Datril
Salicylate	100-250 mcg/mL	>300 mcg/mL	

Continued

Reference Values for Therapeutic Drug Monitoring (cont'd)

Therapeutic Test (Serum) for:	Range	Toxic Levels	Proprietary Test Name(s)
Antineoplastic and Immunosuppressive Medications			
Cyclosporine A	150-350 ng/mL	>400 ng/mL	Sandimmune
Methotrexate (high-dose, 48 hr)	Variable	>1 µmol/L, 48 hr after dose	
Sirolimus (within 1 hr of 2-mg dose)	4.5-14 ng/mL	Variable	Rapamune
Sirolimus (within 1 hr of 5-mg dose)	10-28 ng/mL	Variable	Rapamune
Tacrolimus (FK-506), whole blood	3-20 mcg/L	>15 mcg/L	Prograf
Bronchodilators			
Theophylline (aminophylline)	10-20 mcg/mL	>20 mcg/mL	Theo-Dur
Cardiovascular Medications			
Amiodarone (obtain specimen more than 8 hr after last dose)	1-2 mcg/mL	>2 mcg/mL	Cordarone
Digoxin (specimen must be obtained 12 to 24 hr after last dose)	0.8-2 ng/mL	>2.4 ng/mL	Lanoxin
Disopyramide	2-5 mcg/mL	>7 mcg/mL	Norpace
Flecainide	0.2-1 ng/mL	>1 mcg/mL	Tambocor
Lidocaine	1.5-5 mcg/mL	>6 mcg/mL	Xylocaine
Mexiletine	0.7-2 ng/mL	>2 ng/mL	Mexitil
Procainamide	4-10 mcg/mL	>12 mcg/mL	Pronestyl
Procainamide (measured as procainamide N-acetyl-procainamide)	8-30 mcg/mL	>30 mcg/mL	
Propranolol	50-100 ng/mL	Variable	Inderal
Quinidine	2-5 mcg/mL	>6 mcg/mL	Cardioquin, Quinaglute
Tocainide	4-10 ng/mL	>10 ng/mL	Tonocard
Psychopharmacologic Medications			
Amitriptyline	120-150 ng/mL	>500 ng mL	Elavil, Triavil
Bupropion	25-100 ng/mL	Not applicable	Wellbutrin
Desipramine	150-300 ng/mL	>500 ng/mL	Norpramin
Imipramine	125-250 ng/mL	>400 ng/mL	Tofranil
Lithium (obtain specimen 12 hr after last dose)	0.6-1.5 mEq/L	>1.5 mEq/L	Lithobid
Nortriptyline	50-150 ng/mL	>500 ng/mL	Aventyl, Pamelor

*A peak level may not be done.

Adapted from Bope ET, Kellerman RD: *Conn's current therapy 2012*, Philadelphia, 2012, Saunders.

Therapeutic Monitoring of Anticoagulation Therapy

When the patient is undergoing heparin therapy:

	Normal	Therapeutic Range	Critical Level
Prothrombin time	11.0-12.5 seconds	1.5-2 × normal	
INR	0.8-1.1	2-3	>5.5
Activated partial prothrombin time (aPPT)	30-40 seconds	1.5-2.5 × normal	>70 seconds

■ MEDICATION ADMINISTRATION

Relevant Abbreviations

mL	=	milliliter	PC, pc	=	after meals
fl oz	=	fluid ounce	c̄	=	with
g, Gm, G, GM	=	gram	s̄	=	without
gr	=	grain	Bid, bid	=	twice a day
gtt	=	drop	Tid, tid	=	three times a day
kg	=	kilogram	Qid, qid	=	four times a day
μg, mcg	=	microgram	q4h, q6h, q8h	=	every 4, 6, 8 hours
mEq	=	milliequivalent	PRN	=	whenever necessary
mg	=	milligram	NPO	=	nothing by mouth
l, L	=	liter	STAT	=	immediately
s̄s̄	=	one-half	IM	=	intramuscularly
T, tbsp	=	tablespoon	IV	=	intravenously
t, tsp	=	teaspoon	SubQ	=	subcutaneously
<^	=	less than	SL, subl	=	sublingual
>*	=	greater than	IVPB	=	intravenous
PO, po, os	=	by mouth			piggyback
AC, ac	=	before meals	KVO	=	keep vein open

*Use not recommended.

Adapted from Kee J, Hayes E, McCuistion L: *Pharmacology: a nursing process approach*, ed 8, Philadelphia, 2015, Saunders.

The Joint Commission's Lists of Dangerous Abbreviations, Acronyms, and Symbols

A "minimum list" of dangerous abbreviations, acronyms, and symbols has been approved by The Joint Commission (TJC). The items in Table 5-1 must be included on each accredited organization's "Do Not Use" list.

The Institute for Safe Medication Practices (ISMP) has published a list of dangerous abbreviations (available at http://www.ismp.org) relating to medication use that it recommends should be explicitly prohibited. Two nurses must double-check the following before administration: heparin, insulin, parenteral chemotherapeutic agents, patient-controlled analgesia, and epidural pumps.

The Health Insurance Portability and Accountability Act (HIPAA) privacy requirements state that patient information concerning name, age, diagnosis, and other personal information should not be posted. Charts and medication records must be kept in a confidential area.

TABLE 5-1	The Joint Commission Minimum "Do Not Use" List of Abbreviations	
Do Not Use	**Potential Problem**	**Use Instead**
U (unit)	Mistaken for "0" (zero), "4" (four), or cc	Write "unit"
IU (international unit)	Mistaken for IV (intravenous) or the number 10 (ten)	Write "international unit"
Q.D., QD, q.d., qd (daily)	Mistaken for each other	Write "daily"
Q.O.D., QOD, q.o.d., qod (every other day)	Period after the Q mistaken for "I" and the "O" mistaken for "I"	Write "every other day"
Trailing zero (X.0 mg) [NOTE: Prohibited only for medication-related notations] Lack of leading zero (.X mg)	Decimal point is missed	Never write a zero by itself after a decimal point (X mg), and always use a zero before a decimal point (0.X mg)
MS	Can mean "morphine sulfate" or "magnesium sulfate"	Write "morphine sulfate" or "magnesium sulfate"
MSO_4 and $MgSO_4$	Confused for one another	

The Joint Commission, 2016. Reprinted with permission.

Six Rights of Medication Administration

Right medication. Check the prescriber's order, and check the label with the medication administration record three times.

Right dose. Check the prescriber's order, check the dosage on the medication label three times, and calculate the correct amount to give as per the order.

Right time. Check the prescriber's order, and check the date and time on the medication administration record order three times. Check the expiration date of the medication.

Right route. Check the prescriber's order and verify the route of administration three times on the medication administration record.

Right patient. Check the armband name and number with the medication administration record sheet just before administering the drug, and ask the patient to state his or her name.

Each unit/dose/drug should be checked with the medication administration record, verifying each of the first four rights:

- As the medication is taken from the patient's drawer.
- As the medication is placed, still in its package, in a paper cup or on a small tray.
- Just before opening the package to administer the dose to the patient.

Right documentation. Document the drug **after** it has been given.

Six Responsibilities for Medication Administration

1. Take a complete drug history.
2. Assess the patient for drug allergies.

3. Teach the patient about the drug and side effects to report.
4. Determine the reason the patient is receiving the drug.
5. Be aware of potential interaction with other drugs or foods.
6. Document effect of each drug you administer.

Safety Guidelines to Prevent Medication Errors

When preparing to administer medications:

- Ask yourself why this drug is prescribed for this patient. Know the drug, the patient, and all of the patient's medical conditions.
- Before preparing medications, verify which patients are NPO or off the unit.
- Verify that the medication orders on the medication administration record (MAR)/Kardex have been checked against the prescriber's orders.
- If the patient is a child or an older adult, review the special precautions to be considered.
- Become familiar with the "high alert drug list" from your facility's pharmacy. Be extra careful when administering a drug that is on this list. Be aware of look-alike and sound-alike drugs.
- Become familiar with the list of abbreviations that are no longer to be used, and ask for verification from the prescriber as to what is intended by the abbreviation if it appears in an order.
- Plan ahead, and do not rush when preparing medications for administration.
- Prepare medications for administration in as distraction-free an environment as possible.
- Follow the Six Rights of medication administration every time you prepare and give medications.
- Check each medication with the order thoroughly three times before giving it to the patient.
- Ask before crushing a drug if you do not know whether it can be safely administered after crushing.
- Clarify with the prescriber any illegible writing in a drug order.
- Do not administer a drug if it is not clearly and correctly labeled with name and amount of the drug contained.
- Do not unwrap a unit dose drug before you are at the patient's bedside and ready to administer the medication.
- Check any questionable order or unfamiliar drug or dosage with the pharmacist.
- If an ordered drug dosage seems odd, question it and check the order with the pharmacist or physician.
- Check pertinent laboratory values, and assess for side effects of the drug before giving the next dose.
- If a dosage calculation has to be made for a heart medication, insulin, heparin, or anticancer drug, have the calculation repeated by another nurse and compare the results.
- Review the patient's MAR for any possible drug interactions.
- Determine if the patient is receiving more than one drug with the same action. If so, question the order.
- Ask another nurse to double-check the order and dose you are going to give of any high-risk drug such as IV potassium, heparin, IV cardiac drugs,

insulins, or chemotherapy drugs; both nurses should use the 6 rights. Many agencies require the signature of both nurses.

- Keep the drug in its original container. Discard leftover portions of unused medication from single-dose packages.
- Whenever multiple tablets or vials are needed to prepare a single dose of medication, check with the pharmacist to verify the amount is correct as per the order.
- Become aware of drugs with similar names, and carefully check the original order and why the patient is receiving the drug before administering it.
- Question an excessive dosage increase in a patient's medication.
- Be familiar with every drug you administer. Look it up if you can't remember the information you need to administer it safely.
- Date multiple-dose medication vials as you open them.

At the time of medication administration to the patient:

- Use two patient identifiers. Verify the name and number on the patient's armband with the information on the MAR each time you administer medications to the patient.
- Check the MAR and the chart for noted allergies, and question the patient before administering medications.
- Check each drug at the bedside with the patient's MAR before administering the medication.
- If the patient questions the drug or dose you are about to give, stop and check the situation.
- Sign that a medication has been given only after the patient has received it.
- Do not leave a medication dose at the patient's bedside.
- Document only after the patient has actually taken the medication.

When working with the patient for error prevention:

- Teach the patient about the drugs he or she is taking and the importance of proper identification of the medication before it is taken.
- Familiarize the patient with the color and shape of each medication, but consider that generic forms of the drug may differ. Instruct the patient to ask the pharmacist if a refill looks different from the last one.
- Obtain a complete drug history from the patient, including herbals, over-the-counter medications, and supplements.

If a medication error occurs, always report it!

Check Those Lab Tests!

When preparing to administer medications, you should know the laboratory test values relative to the action or potential adverse effects of each drug. For some drugs you will be checking to see if the medication is effective; for others, checking indicates if the drug is at a therapeutic level in the patient's body. Many drugs can affect kidney function, liver function, or bone marrow and blood cell function; laboratory tests are checked to verify whether adverse effects are occurring. Checking your patient's lab values first thing during the shift will save you time later. You will not always find the laboratory test data you are seeking, but it is your responsibility to check. Become familiar with the laboratory test values that should be checked when giving various medications. Here is a list of common medications, or types of medications, and the test values to be checked. This is not a complete list. Check your drug handbook for other specific test values that should be checked for a particular medication.

Medication	Laboratory Test Value to Check
Digoxin (Lanoxin)	Serum digoxin; K^+
Lasix	K^+
Procainamide	Serum level
Heparin	aPTT
Warfarin (Coumadin)	INR, PT
Antibiotics	CBC, liver function, renal function
Tobramycin	Serum peak and trough levels
Gentamicin	Liver functions—AST, ALT, bilirubin
Vancomycin	Kidney functions—BUN, creatinine
Chloramphenicol	LDH, alkaline phosphatase
Amikacin	Therapeutic level; BUN, creatinine
Anticonvulsants	Specific drug serum level, CBC, AST, ALT, bilirubin, BUN, creatinine
Theophylline, aminophylline	Serum theophylline level (bronchodilators)
Albuterol	ABGs
Antihypertensives	CBC, electrolytes
NSAIDs, acetaminophen, ibuprofen	CBC, liver functions—AST, ALT; kidney functions—BUN, creatinine
Hypoglycemics, insulins	Serum glucose, finger-stick glucose
Cortisone, corticosteroids	K^+, CBC, serum glucose
Cholesterol-lowering statins	Cholesterol, HDL, LDL, triglycerides, AST, ALT, CPK
Iron preparations	CBC, HgB, Hct

Choosing the Correct Needle Size

The larger the number of the gauge, the smaller the needle.

For	Use
Intradermal Injections	
Intradermal skin test	27 gauge, $\frac{1}{2}$ in
Subcutaneous Injections	
Allergy injection	27 gauge, $\frac{1}{2}$ in or $\frac{3}{8}$ in
Immunization (some)	25 gauge, $\frac{3}{8}$ in
Intramuscular Injections	
Thin solutions	23-25 gauge, 1 to $1\frac{1}{2}$ in*
Antibiotic	22 gauge, 1 to $1\frac{1}{2}$ in*
Oil-based solution	21 gauge, 1 to $1\frac{1}{2}$ in*

*Length depends on size of patient and the injection site chosen; larger patients need a longer needle to reach the proper depth.

Sites for Intramuscular (IM) and Subcutaneous (Subcut) Injections

Avoid the dorsogluteal site whenever possible. The risk of hitting the sciatic nerve is great in this area and it is not a recommended site.

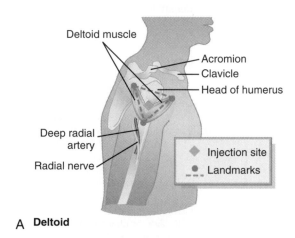

A **Deltoid**

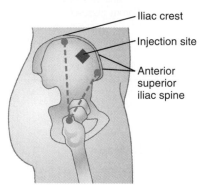

B **Ventrogluteal**

Sites for Intramuscular (IM) and Subcutaneous (Subcut) Injections (cont'd)

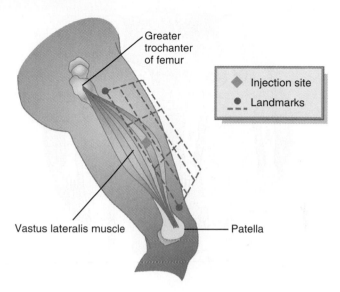

C **Vastus Lateralis**

Clinical Quick Reference

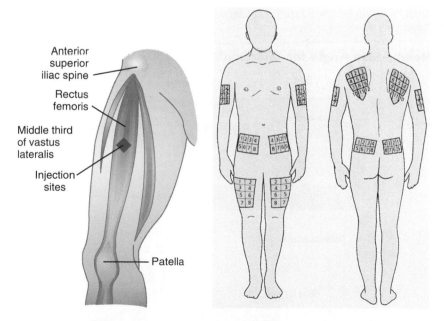

D **Rectus Femoris**   E Subcutaneous Rotation Sites

(From Kee J, Hayes E, McCuistion L: *Pharmacology: a nursing process approach,* ed 8, Philadelphia, 2015, Saunders.)

Common Sites for Intradermal Injections

Forearm is most common.

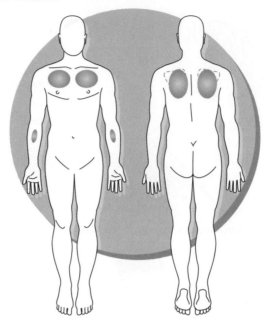

(From Kee J, Hayes E, McCuistion L: *Pharmacology: a nursing process approach,* ed 8, Philadelphia, 2015, Saunders.)

Needle-Skin Angle for Injection

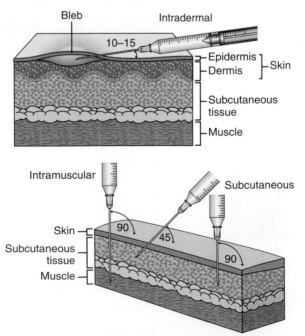

(From Kee J, Hayes E, McCuistion L: *Pharmacology: a nursing process approach,* ed 8, Philadelphia, 2015, Saunders.)

Dosage and Solution Calculation Formulas

BASIC DRUG CALCULATIONS FORMULA

$$\frac{D\,(\text{desired})}{H\,(\text{on hand})} \times V\,(\text{vehicle, drug from})$$

Example:

Order: amoxicillin 100 mg PO q6h
Available: amoxicillin 250 mg/5 mL

$$\frac{D}{H} \times = \frac{100\ \text{mg}}{250\ \text{mg}} \times 5\ \text{mL}$$

$$= \frac{500}{250} = 2\ \text{mL amoxicillin}$$

RATIO AND PROPORTION

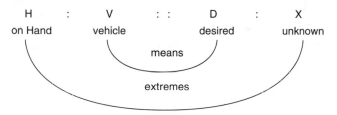

Example:

Order: amoxicillin 100 mg PO q6h
Available: amoxicillin 250 mg/5 mL

$$
\begin{array}{cccccccc}
H & : & V & : : & D & : & X \\
250\ \text{mg} & : & 5\ \text{mL} & : : & 100\ \text{mg} & : & X\ \text{mL}
\end{array}
$$

$$250\,X = 500$$
$$X = 2\ \text{mL amoxicillin}$$

BODY WEIGHT (KILOGRAMS)

To change pounds to kilograms, divide by 2.2.
Example: Change 44 pounds to kg

$$44 \div 2.2 = 20\ \text{kg}$$
$$\text{Dosage/kg/day} = \text{dosage/day}$$
$$(\text{Dosage} \times \text{kg} = \text{dose/day})$$

Example:
Order: drug 6 mg/kg/day in four divided doses

$$6\ \text{mg} \times 20\ \text{kg} \times 1\ \text{day} = 120\ \text{mg/day}$$
$$120 \div 4 = 30\ \text{mg per dose}$$

From Kee J, Hayes E, McCuistion L: *Pharmacology: a nursing process approach*, ed 8, Philadelphia, 2015, Saunders.

Major Drug Categories by Generic Name Endings

Generic Name Ending	Example(s)	Type of Drug	Common Action
-pril	Lisinopril	Angiotensin-converting enzyme (ACE) inhibitor	Antihypertensive that relaxes arterial vessels
-sartan	Losartan	Angiotensin-receptor blocker	Antihypertensive that blocks action of vasoconstriction effects of angiotensin II
-olol, -alol, and -ilol	Atenolol, labetalol, carvedilol	Beta blocker	Antihypertensive/antianginal that blocks beta-adrenergic receptors in vascular smooth muscle
-statin	Atorvastatin	Antilipemic	Inhibits HMG-CoA reductase enzyme, thereby reducing cholesterol synthesis
-dipine	Amlodipine	Peripheral vessel calcium channel blocker	Antihypertensive/antianginal that produces relaxation of coronary smooth muscle and vascular smooth muscle; dilates coronary arteries
-afril	Sildenafil	Erectile agent	Peripheral vasodilator that promotes a penile erection
-floxacin	Ciprofloxacin	Broad-spectrum antiinfective	Inhibits bacteria by interfering with DNA
-prazole	Esomeprazole	Proton pump inhibitor	Suppresses gastric secretions, preventing gastric reflux and gastric and duodenal ulcers
-tidine	Famotidine	Block histamine-2 (H_2) receptor	Inhibits histamine at H_2-receptor sites, decreasing gastric secretions
-azole	Fluconazole	Antifungal	Causes direct damage to fungal membrane
-cyclovir	Acyclovir	Antiherpetic	Interferes with DNA synthesis, causing decreased viral replication
-pam	Diazepam	Antianxiolytic	Central nervous system (CNS) depression
-mycin	Garamycin	Aminoglycoside antibiotic	Bactericidal
ceph-	Cephalexin	Cephalosporin antibiotic	Cell lysis or cell death
-thromycin	Azithromycin	Macrolide antibiotic	Bacteriostatic or bacteriocidal
-cillin	Ampicillin	Penicillin antibiotic	Inhibits synthesis of cell wall
-cycline	Doxycycline	Tetracycline antibiotic	Inhibits protein synthesis of bacteria

Major Drug Categories by Generic Name Endings (cont'd)

Generic Name Ending	Example(s)	Type of Drug	Common Action
-arin	Heparin, warfarin	Anticoagulant	Blocks conversion of thrombin and fibrinogen to fibrin
-azosin	Terazosin	Antihypertensive	Inhibits sympathetic vasoconstriction
-vin	Vincristin	Antineoplastic	Causes metaphase arrest
-dopa	Sinemet	Antiparkinsonian agent	Replaces dopamine
-azine	Thorazine	Antipsychotic agent	Depresses cerebral cortex
-cyclovir	Acyclovir	Antiviral agent	Interferes with viral DNA synthesis
-dronate	Fosamax	Bone resorption inhibitor	Decreases rate of bone resorption
-tropium	Spiriva	Bronchodilator	Relaxes bronchial smooth muscle
-phylline	Aminophylline	Respiratory smooth muscle relaxer	Produces bronchodilation; exact mechanism unknown
-oxin	Digoxin	Cardiac glycoside	Increases cardiac output and force of contraction; decreases heart rate
-fate	Carafate	Cytoprotective agent	Adheres to peptic ulcer site and absorbs pepsin
-sone	Prednisone	Steroid	Decreases inflammation

Adapted from a presentation by Barb Bancroft at the California Vocational Nurse Educators Conference in Sacramento, CA, April 25, 2008.

High-Alert Medications

The following drugs can be dangerous if given in error. Be especially careful when administering these drugs. Be certain that there is a patient indication for the drug; that you are aware of the action, side effects, and adverse effects of the drug; and that you have assessed for those effects before giving the next dose. Check pertinent lab values before giving the drug. For cardiac drugs, check vital sign parameters to ensure safe administration.

- Amphotericin B, IV
- Antiepileptic drugs, injection, IV
- Antipsychotic drugs, injection
- Cardiac drugs, IV
- Chemotherapy agents
- Corticosteroid drugs, oral, injection, IV
- Dextrose, hypertonic solution IV
- Epinephrine, injection, IV
- Epoprostenol (Flolan), IV
- Heparin, low-molecular-weight heparin
- Insulin, subcutaneous, IV*
- Lasix, IV
- Lidocaine, IV
- Magnesium sulfate, injection

- Methotrexate, oral, use other than for oncology patients
- Narcotic drugs, oral, injection, IV
- Norepinephrine, IV
- Opium, tincture
- Oxytocin, IV
- Nitroprusside sodium, injection
- Oral hypoglycemic drugs
- Potassium chloride, injection
- Potassium phosphates, injection
- Promethazine, IV
- Sedative drugs, injection, IV
- Sodium chloride injection, greater than 0.9% concentration
- Sterile water for injection in vials larger than 100 mL
- Total parenteral nutrition solutions

*Insulin doses should always be checked with another nurse after the dose is drawn up and before it is administered.

Insulins

TYPES AND ACTIONS

Preparation	Brand Name	Onset (hr)	Peak (hr)	Duration (hr)
Rapid Acting				
Insulin aspart injection	NovoLog	0.25	1-3	3-5
Insulin lispro injection	Humalog	0.25	0.5-1.5	3-4
Insulin glulisine injection	Apidra	0.3	0.5-1.5	5
Short Acting				
Regular human insulin injection	Humulin R	0.5	2-4	6-8
	Novolin R, ReliOn	0.5	2.5-5	8
Intermediate Acting				
Human insulin isophane	Humulin N	1.5	4-12	24
suspension NPH	Novulin N	3-4	6-12	12-18
Insulin zinc suspension (Lente)	ReliOn N	1.5	4-12	24
Humulin R (Concentrated U-500)	Novolin L, Humulin R (U-500)	1	6-8	5.7-24
Insulin detemir injection		1	6-8	5.7-2.4
Long Acting				
Insulin glargine injection	Lantus* Levemir	2-4	None	24
Combination Insulin				
70% Insulin aspart protamine suspension/30% insulin aspart injection	NovoLog Mix 70/30	0.25	1-4	24
75% Insulin lispro protamine suspension/25% insulin lispro injection	Humalog Mix 75/25, Humalog Mix 50/50	0.25	1-4	24

TYPES AND ACTIONS (cont'd)

Preparation	Brand Name	Onset (hr)	Peak (hr)	Duration (hr)
70% Human insulin isophane suspension (NPH)/30% human insulin injection (regular)	Humulin 70/30 Novolin 70/30 ReliOn/Novolin 70/30	0.5	2-12	24
50% Human insulin isophane suspension (NPH)/50% human insulin injection (regular)	Humulin 50/50	0.5	3-5	24
75% Insulin lispro protamine/ 25% insulin lispro	Humalog 75/25	0.25	1-2	24

*Never mix Lantus with any other insulin.
Adapted from Ignatavicius DD, Workman ML: *Medical-surgical nursing: critical thinking for collaborative care*, ed 7, Philadelphia, 2013, Saunders.

HYPOGLYCEMIA VERSUS HYPERGLYCEMIA

	Hypoglycemia (<60 mg/dL)	Hyperglycemia (>250 mg/dL)
Cause	Too much insulin Skipped or delayed meals Too much exercise	Too little insulin Overeating Emotional stress Illness, infection, stroke, heart attack, pregnancy
Early symptoms	Sweating, shaking, weakness Headache, dizziness Hunger	Excessive thirst Frequent urination Fatigue, weakness
Late symptoms	Numbness of lips or tongue Difficulty concentrating Irritability, mood changes Blurred vision, pallor If untreated: seizures, coma	Nausea, vomiting, abdominal pain Flushed, dry skin Fruity breath, drowsiness, lethargy Loss of appetite, general aching If untreated: labored breathing, coma, ketoacidosis

Adapted from *Mosby's PDQ for LPN*, ed 3, St Louis, 2013, Mosby.

GUIDELINES FOR INSULIN ADMINISTRATION
* Check all insulin orders with the physician's order sheet.
* Verify the patient's current blood glucose level per glucometer reading or lab work. Assess the patient for signs of hyperglycemia or hypoglycemia. Symptoms of **hyperglycemia** include nausea; vomiting; abdominal cramps; fatigue; increased thirst; increased urination; increased hunger followed by anorexia; weakness; dry mouth; acetone breath; and rapid, deep respirations. Signs of **hypoglycemia** include sweating; cold, clammy skin; feelings of numbness in fingers in toes and around mouth; rapid heartbeat; headache; nervousness; shakiness; faintness; slurred speech; hunger; vision changes; unsteady gait; weakness.
* Obtain permission to recheck blood sugar level by glucometer.

- Administer insulin as close to the time ordered as possible, but consider when a meal will be served.
- Gently roll and invert the bottle to mix and ensure even drug particle distribution before withdrawing the solution from the vial.
- Check date on vial to be certain the insulin is in-date.
- When mixing regular and long-acting insulin, put air into the long-acting insulin vial and then put air into the regular insulin and draw up the correct amount of the regular insulin; draw up the exact amount of the long-acting insulin last.
- Always have another nurse verify the type and dosage of each insulin ordered as you prepare the injection.
- Use only an insulin syringe (insulin syringes are measured in units of insulin).
- Inject at a 45- to 60-degree angle.
- Rotate injection sites to prevent lipodystrophy. Do not massage the site after injection. Use one site area daily for 1 week and then rotate to a new site. Keep a record of injection sites. Sites within an area should be $1\frac{1}{2}$ inches apart. Abdominal sites are preferred for consistent absorption.
- If the patient gives his or her own insulin at home and is able to administer it in the hospital, allow the opportunity to do so.
- Never give any type but regular insulin by IV infusion.
- Watch for signs of hypoglycemia around the time that the insulin given is expected to peak (see the "Types and Actions" section under "Insulins" in this chapter). Give an oral carbohydrate snack if symptoms occur and blood glucose reading is low. Milk and crackers or 4 ounces of orange juice are commonly given. If available, protein in the snack is best.
- Report hypoglycemic reactions to the staff nurse and your instructor immediately.
- Remember that only regular insulin can be given IV.
- Continue to monitor the patient.
- Teach how to use an insulin pen if that is to be the mode of insulin delivery:
  - Screw on a new needle.
  - If pen requires priming to remove air, follow directions for priming.
  - Turn the dial knob on the end of the pen to the correct number of units.
  - Insert the needle under the skin.
  - Press the button on the end of the pen.
  - Count to five before removing the needle from the skin.

Digitalis Therapy

Digitalis is given to strengthen myocardial muscle action and slow the heart rate. Drug toxicity occurs frequently with this drug. **Early signs of toxicity** include anorexia, diarrhea, headache, confusion, fatigue, irritability, drowsiness, halos around lights, and green or yellow vision. **Further signs of toxicity** include cardiac arrhythmia, particularly bradycardia, depression, and convulsion. **A below-normal level of serum potassium predisposes the patient to digitalis toxicity.**

NURSING CONSIDERATIONS

- Auscultate the apical pulse for 60 seconds to detect changes in rate or rhythm.
- If the heart rate is less than 60 or more than 100 beats/min, check the physician's orders for a notation as to whether the dose should be given or

whether it should be withheld until the physician has been notified. Assess for other signs of toxicity before calling the physician (dose is held if toxicity is present).
- Check the last laboratory test level of digitalis and the last serum potassium level before administering the dose. Assess for signs of hypokalemia: muscle weakness, fatigue, anorexia, confusion, weak pulse and nausea.
- Assess total medication regimen to determine possible interactions of digitalis with other drugs.
- If the patient is taking both digitalis and a diuretic that is not potassium sparing, potassium supplementation should be administered.

PATIENT TEACHING
- Digitalis preparations should be taken at the same time each day.
- Check the pulse for a full minute before taking each dose.
- Report signs of digitalis toxicity; pay attention to early signs.
- Report any new irregular rhythm or abnormal pulse rate to the physician.
- Watch for signs of potassium depletion (hypokalemia). Teach the signs.
- Do not skip doses of the prescribed potassium supplement.
- If a digitalis dose is missed, do not take an extra dose without consulting the physician.
- Keep follow-up appointments with the physician.

Steroid (Cortisone) Therapy
- Once-a-day steroid doses are given between 7:00 AM and 8:00 AM for best results, because this is when the body normally releases these hormones.
- Check for possible interactions with other drugs the patient is receiving.
- Insulin dosages may have to be adjusted when the patient is receiving steroids.
- Administer oral steroids with food or milk to minimize gastric irritation.
- Patients who are on NPO status and are receiving parenteral steroids should be monitored for gastric bleeding. Medications to protect the gastric mucosa are usually given concurrently.
- Do not omit steroid dosages. If a dose has been inadvertently skipped, consult the physician.
- If the patient has been receiving steroids for 1 week or longer, the dosage must be tapered slowly rather than discontinued abruptly.
- Observe for infection, and protect the patient from exposure to infection while receiving steroids. Steroids can mask infection and sometimes suppress the immune system.
- Assess for potassium imbalances and glucose imbalances.
- Increase calcium intake. Teach the patient receiving long-term steroid therapy measures to help prevent osteoporosis.
- Encourage regular eye examinations when the patient is receiving long-term therapy; steroids can cause cataracts and glaucoma.
- Assess for Cushing's syndrome symptoms: moon face, buffalo hump, hirsutism, and edema.
- Observe for side effects of steroid therapy: nausea, abdominal pain, hypertension, pathologic fractures, osteoporosis, delayed wound healing, headache, mood changes, insomnia, and dizziness on standing.

Clinical Quick Reference

Anticoagulant Therapy

Your patient may receive heparin by continuous IV infusion, intermittent IV injection, or subcutaneous injection. Consider the following points:

- Protamine sulfate is the antidote for heparin overdose and should be kept on hand on the unit.
- The effectiveness of heparin therapy is judged by the extension of usual clotting time to 2.0 to 2.5 times normal (approximately 60 to 70 seconds). The activated partial thromboplastin time (aPTT) or partial thromboplastin time (PTT) is used to determine the clotting time. The result should be no more than 2.0 to 2.5 times the control time. The test should be done before therapy is begun and then monitored periodically, depending on how much heparin the patient is receiving and whether it is being given IV or by injection.
- **All heparin dosages should be checked with another nurse as they are prepared.**
- Heparin subcutaneous injections are given in the abdominal fat at least 2 inches from the umbilicus in the area between the iliac crests.
- Enoxaparin (Lovenox) is a low-molecular-weight heparin for injection that is widely used. Frequent blood tests are not required with this medication.
- Do not aspirate before injecting the heparin, because aspiration causes tissue trauma and bruising.
- Wait 10 to 15 seconds after injecting before removing the needle.
- Do not massage the area, because massaging causes increased bruising.
- Ice may be applied for 5 minutes to prevent bruising if this is a problem for the patient.
- Rotate the injection site from side to side.
- The patient receiving heparin by continuous IV infusion should be placed on a special mattress to decrease bruising.
- Monitor the patient closely for signs of increased bleeding or hemorrhage, such as bloody urine (hematuria); dark, tarry stools (melena); bleeding of surgical wounds; bleeding gums; nosebleeds (epistaxis); hematomas; bloody sputum; bruising (ecchymosis); increased vaginal bleeding; neurologic changes; and signs and symptoms of hypovolemic shock.
- Patients who have been treated with heparin are often started on warfarin sodium (Coumadin) orally before the heparin is discontinued. This is done because it takes 3 days for the warfarin levels in the blood to build up to an effective anticoagulant level.
- Warfarin therapy's effectiveness is judged by the prothrombin time (PT) test. The result should be no more than 2.0 to 2.5 times the control value (usually 12 to 14 seconds). Prothrombin time international normalized ratio (INR) is therapeutic from 2.0 to 3.5. When intracoronary stents or recurrent systemic emboli are treated with warfarin, the INR is kept between 3.0 and 4.5. If an INR test is not available, the prothrombin time (PT) test is done. The result should be no more than 2.0 to 2.5 times the control value (usually 12 to 13 seconds).
- The antidote for warfarin overdosage is vitamin K by injection.
- Patients may also be started on antiplatelet aggregation medications such as clopidogrel (Plavix), aspirin, ticlopidine (Ticlid), dipyridamole (Persantine), dabigatran (Pradaxa), or ticagrelor (Brilinta).

PATIENT TEACHING

- Do not take aspirin, nonsteroidal antiinflammatory drugs (NSAIDs), or other salicylates while receiving anticoagulants.
- Avoid situations that could cause injury and bleeding, including contact sports. An electric razor may be used rather than a safety razor. Use a soft toothbrush, and avoid vigorous nose blowing.
- Many medications interact with warfarin; consult the physician regarding the possible interaction with other medications and supplements.
- Keep the amount of green vegetables containing vitamin K consistent in the diet.
- Limit alcohol intake.
- Take the medication at the same time each day.
- Inform all physicians and dentists that you are taking an anticoagulant.
- Wear an ID band stating that an anticoagulant is being taken.
- If bleeding occurs, apply pressure for 5 to 10 minutes and call the physician.
- Schedule follow-up tests to determine the effect of anticoagulant therapy.

■ INTRAVENOUS THERAPY

Calculating Intravenous Flow Rates

INTRAVENOUS FLOW RATE: CONTINUOUS—METHOD I

Amount of fluid ÷ hours to administer = mL/hr:

$$\frac{\text{mL/hr} \times \text{gtts/mL (IV set)}}{60 \text{ min/hr}} = \text{gtts/min}$$

Example:
Order: 1000 mL, D_5 ½; NS in 8 hr
IV set: macrodrip, 10 gtt/mL
1000 mL ÷ 8 hr = 125 mL/hr

$$\frac{125 \text{ mL/h} \times \overset{1}{\cancel{10}} \text{ gtts/mL}}{\underset{6}{\cancel{60}} \text{ min/hr}} = 21 \text{ gtts/min}$$

INTRAVENOUS FLOW RATE: INTERMITTENT—VOLUMETRIC PUMP

$$\text{Amount of solution} \div \frac{\text{Min to administer}}{60 \text{ min/hr}} = \text{mL/hr}$$

Example:
Order: 5 mL of drug solution in 100 mL of D_5W in 45 min

$$105 \text{ mL} \div \frac{45 \text{ min}}{60 \text{ min/hr}} \text{ (invert divisor and multiply)}$$

$$= 105 \times \frac{\overset{4}{\cancel{60}}}{\underset{3}{\cancel{45}}} = 140 \text{ mL/hr}$$

Volumetric pump: 140 mL/hr to deliver 105 mL in 45 min.

INTRAVENOUS FLOW RATE: INTERMITTENT—SECONDARY SETS: BURETROL AND ADD-A-LINE

$$\frac{\text{Amount of solution} \times \text{gtts/mL (set)}}{\text{Min to administer}} = \text{gtts/min}$$

Example:
Order: 5 mL drug solution in 50 mL of D_5W in 30 min
IV set: Buretrol (60 gtt/mL)

$$\frac{55 \text{ mL} \times \overset{2}{\cancel{60}} \text{ gtts}}{\underset{1}{\cancel{30}} \text{ min}} = 110 \text{ gtts/min}$$

INTRAVENOUS FLOW RATE: CONTINUOUS—METHOD II

$$\frac{\text{Amount of fluid} \times \text{gtts/mL (IV set)}}{\text{H to administer} \times \text{min/h (60)}} = \text{gtts/min}$$

Example:
Order: 1000 mL of D_5W in 10 hr
IV set: microdrip, 60 gtt/mL

$$\frac{\overset{100}{\cancel{1000}} \text{ mL} \times \overset{1}{\cancel{60}} \text{ gtts/mL}}{\underset{1}{\cancel{10}} \text{ h} \times \underset{1}{\cancel{60}} \text{ min/h}} = 100 \text{ gtts/min}$$

From Kee J, Hayes E, McCuistion L: *Pharmacology: a nursing process approach*, ed 8, Philadelphia, 2015, Saunders.

Intravenous Flow Rate Chart

Administration Sets Delivering 10 gtt/mL

Amount to be infused (mL)	1000	1000	1000	1000
Time of infusion (hours)	12	10	8	6
Rate of flow (gtt/min)	14	17	21	28

Administration Sets Delivering 15 gtt/mL

Amount to be infused (mL)	1000	1000	1000	1000
Time of infusion (hours)	12	10	8	6
Rate of flow (gtt/min)	21	25	31	42

Administration Sets Delivering 20 gtt/mL

Amount to be infused (mL)	1000	1000	1000	1000
Time of infusion (hours)	12	10	8	6
Rate of flow (gtt/min)	28	33	42	56

Microdrip Administration Sets Delivering 60 gtt/mL

Amount to be infused (mL)	250	250	500	1000
Time of infusion (hours)	24	12	12	24
Rate of flow (gtt/min)	10	21	42	42

Intravenous Flow Rate Chart (cont'd)

Administration Sets Delivering 10 gtt/mL

Amount to be infused (mL)	50	50	50
Time of infusion (minutes)	20	30	60
Rate of flow (gtt/min)	25	17	8

Administration Sets Delivering 15 gtt/mL

Amount to be infused (mL)	50	50	50
Time of infusion (hours)	20	30	60
Rate of flow (gtt/min)	38	25	12

Administration Sets Delivering 20 gtt/mL

Amount to be infused (mL)	50	50	50
Time of infusion (minutes)	20	30	60
Rate of flow (gtt/min)	50	33	17

Administration Sets Delivering 60 gtt/mL (Microdrip)

Amount to be infused (mL)	50	100	250
Time of infusion (hours)	2	8	6
Rate of flow (gtt/min)	25	12	42

Calculation of Intravenous Intake

Start with the amount that was in the IV container at the beginning of the shift. If that entire amount infuses and a new container is hung, note the amount that is infused from the old container on the shift intake and output (I&O) sheet under "IV intake."

Next, at the end of the shift, note how much of the solution in the new container hung during the shift has infused. Draw a line and initial it with the time at that point on the container. Write the amount infused on the shift I&O sheet under "IV intake." Add the two amounts together to obtain the total IV intake for the shift.

To calculate the amount left to count in the IV container (for the next shift), subtract the amount infused from the new container from the total volume hung.

Example:

	Count	Infused
Count at beginning of shift	450 mL	—
New solution added at 11:30 AM	1000 mL	450 mL
Amount infused at 2:00 PM	—	325 mL
Amount left to count at end of shift	675 mL	—
Total amount of IV intake	—	775 mL

Intake from IV Pump

Rate × time in hours = mL intake	100 mL/hr × 24 hr	2400 mL
Volume of medication × # of doses = mL intake	165 mL × 4 doses	660 mL
Flush volume × # of flushes	30 mL × 6	180 mL
Total amount of IV intake	—	***3240 mL***

Intravenous Site Placement

- Identify suitable vein for placement of IV catheter or needle. The cephalic, basilic, and median cubital veins are preferred in adults (Figure 5-7).

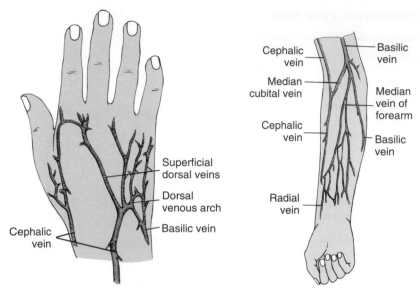

FIGURE 5-7 Veins for intravenous (IV) site placement. (From Perry AG, Potter PA, Elkin MK: *Nursing interventions and clinical skills,* ed 5, St Louis, 2011, Mosby.)

- Use the most distal site in the nondominant arm, if possible. Choose a site that will least interfere with activities of daily living (ADLs).
- Clip arm hair with clippers and a sterile disposable head if site has considerable hair.
- Place extremity in dependent position if possible.
- Using a sterile IV start kit, place the tourniquet 4 to 6 inches above the chosen site. Do not apply tourniquet too tightly; check for radial pulse, indicating good blood flow distal to the tourniquet.
- Release tourniquet temporarily and prepare all equipment. Replace the tourniquet when ready to perform the puncture.
- Measures to increase venous distention include lightly tapping over the vein, stroking the extremity from distal to proximal below the proposed venipuncture site, having the patient open and close the fist and then leaving it closed, applying moistened warm washcloth to site for several minutes, and dangling the extremity for several minutes.
- Follow correct procedure for cleansing the site and inserting the catheter or needle. Always wear latex or blood-impermeable gloves when inserting an IV catheter or needle.

Characteristics of Commonly Used Intravenous Fluids

Solution	Tonicity	Calories	Use
0.9% Normal saline (NS)	Isotonic	0	Fluid replacement, treatment of metabolic acidosis in presence of fluid loss, correction of sodium depletion; used before and after blood transfusion

Characteristics of Commonly Used Intravenous Fluids (cont'd)

Solution	Tonicity	Calories	Use
0.45% Normal saline (½ NS)	Hypotonic	0	Electrolyte replacement of sodium and chloride
5% Dextrose in water (D₅W)	Isotonic	170	Treatment of hypovolemia
10% Dextrose in water (D₁₀W)	Hypertonic	340	Nutrient and electrolyte replacement
5% Dextrose in 0.9% saline (D₅NS 0.9%)	Hypertonic	170	Treatment of circulatory insufficiency; fluid replacement
5% Dextrose in 0.45% saline (D₅ ½ NS)	Hypertonic	170	Maintenance of body fluids with nutrients and for treatment of fluid volume deficit
10% Dextrose in 0.9% saline (D₁₀NS 0.9%)	Hypertonic	340	Nutrient and electrolyte replacement (sodium and chloride)
Hartmann's solution	Isotonic	0	Extracellular fluid replacement for loss due to vomiting, diarrhea, or severe diuresis
5% Dextrose in lactated Ringer's solution (D₅RL)	Hypertonic	170	Electrolyte replacement plus nutrient
Lactated Ringer's solution	Isotonic	0	Replaces sodium without increasing chloride levels

Setting up a "Piggyback" Minibag Medication

1. Check the medication with the order.
2. Verify that the medication is compatible with the main IV solution and its additives plus any other infusion connected to the IV line.
3. Remove the secondary (piggyback) tubing from its package, and close the roller clamp.
4. Spike the piggyback medication container.
5. Squeeze the drip chamber and open the roller clamp to prime the tubing, keeping the connector sterile; close the roller clamp.
6. Recheck the medication with the order or medication administration record (MAR).
7. Label the tubing with the date and time.
8. Take the medication to the patient and perform the third medication check, verifying the patient identification and correct time.
9. Verify the patient's allergies and that there is no allergy to the piggyback medication.
10. Assess for side effects of a previous dose of the same medication. If adverse effects have occurred, withhold the medication and notify the physician.
11. Hang the piggyback minibag medication on the other arm of the IV pole.
12. Lower the main IV container using the hanger that came with the secondary tubing set.
13. Cleanse the highest Y-site injection port below the drip chamber on the administration set tubing.
14. Attach the secondary tubing to the Y-site injection port.
15. Open the roller clamp on the secondary set, and regulate the flow to the desired rate.

To set up the piggyback on the infusion pump:
Remember that the setting on the infusion pump is in mL/hr. Use the secondary screen (button for PB or "secondary") to program the proper flow rate after calculating it. Enter the volume to be infused and the rate of infusion in mL/hr. Hang the piggyback higher than the primary bag of fluid. Follow the instructions for the brand of pump used in the facility. If in doubt, ask your staff nurse or your instructor to check the setting. Check the compatibility of the piggyback medication with all other fluids and meds flowing in the main line (patient-controlled analgesia [PCA] medication, primary bag medications, etc.). Consider whether the combined rate of flow is safe for the patient.

16. Chart the medication.
17. Return when the time for the piggyback medication to infuse has ended.
18. Remove the secondary set and empty the piggyback container.
19. Raise the primary IV container and re-regulate the flow to the ordered rate.
20. Discard the empty piggyback container appropriately.
21. Note the amount of the piggyback medication that infused on the intake and output (I&O) sheet.

Intravenous Drug Compatibility

Any time an IV drug is to be given by IV **push** injection into an existing IV line or by IV piggyback, compatibility with the solution that is infusing and any other drugs being infused must be checked before administration. Reasons for this caution are as follows:

- A physical incompatibility may occur. For example, when phenytoin (Dilantin) is injected into an IV line containing dextrose, a white precipitate forms, clogging the line.
- A chemical incompatibility may occur where one drug inactivates the other, making it ineffective.
- Dilantin is never injected into any solution other than saline.
- Actions to be taken before IV drug administration, in addition to the following Six Rights and Responsibilities, include:
  1. Checking an IV compatibility chart or a drug handbook.
  2. Calling the pharmacist for information on compatibility.
  3. Verifying that the solution used to dilute the drug for an IV piggyback is compatible with the drug.
  4. Flushing the IV line with a compatible solution before and after administering the drug.
  5. **Administering the drug at the recommended rate for a bolus injection to prevent speed shock.**
  6. Correctly flushing an intermittent IV cannula before and after administering a drug. The flush is injected at the same rate as the bolus.

Intravenous Pumps: Tips for Use and Troubleshooting

- IV pumps vary greatly by manufacturer; obtain assistance as needed to learn the specific features.
- Check the medication, calculate the correct dosage, and determine the pump setting prior to entering the patient's room.
- For adult use, most pumps will deliver mL/hr. Set the pump for the correct rate in mL/hr.

- Pumps usually allow you to set a total volume; the machine's alarm will sound when it reaches that volume. (Use this feature to call you back at the end of the infusion or sooner as needed according to your clinical judgment.)
- Before you leave the room, check to ensure the following:
  - Patient is comfortable and there is no swelling or redness at the insertion site.
  - Appropriate clamps are open.
  - Intermittent dripping (not continuous) is observed in the drip chamber.
- Pumps can malfunction; assessment of site and equipment every 1 to 2 hours is a typical hospital policy.
- If the IV pump is continually alarming:
  - Check IV site for infiltration, clotting, etc.
  - Check tubing for kinks or air.
  - Check clamps and flow regulators.
  - Check IV bag to see whether there is fluid for infusion.
  - Make sure the pump is plugged into an electrical source.
  - Recheck settings on the pump.
  - Change the position of the patient's extremity (the IV may be positional).
  - Try turning the pump off and resetting it. Try another pump.

From deWit SC, O'Neill P: *Fundamental concepts and skills for nursing*, ed 4, Philadelphia, 2014, Saunders.

Guidelines for Monitoring a Blood Transfusion

Students are not allowed to administer blood products but are often asked to monitor the patient who is receiving a blood transfusion. The student should accompany the nurse through each step of the process to become familiar with the procedure and the safeguards used when administering blood products.

NURSING CONSIDERATIONS

- Double-check the physician's order.
- Verify that a consent form for blood administration has been signed.
- Assess to determine whether the patient has ever had a transfusion reaction.
- Administer any medications ordered to prevent transfusion reaction (e.g., antipyretic, antihistamine, or steroid).
- Verify that the correct size of IV cannula is in place. An 18-gauge cannula is preferable for trauma patients; a 20-gauge or 22-gauge may be used for some blood products.
- Use a Y-type blood administration set of tubing with a filter. The blood container is attached to one side of the Y, and a container of normal saline is attached to the other side of the Y.
- **Before the container of blood is attached to the patient, the label is checked with the blood bracelet and ID band on the patient by two nurses.** Two identifiers are used, such as patient name and hospital ID number. These identifiers verify that the correct patient, blood type, and unit match the patient's blood. The numbers must match between the blood container and blood band on the patient's arm. The ID check should include the following:
  - The patient's full name (check armband and ask the patient)
  - Patient's hospital number
  - Blood unit number
  - Blood group, Rh factor, and ABO designation

- Expiration date
- Type and crossmatch number
- Baseline vital signs, including temperature, are taken just before the blood transfusion is started.
- Use only saline (0.9% NaCl) before or during the transfusion in the same IV tubing. Start the saline slowly, before the blood arrives from the blood bank.
- Blood infusions must be started within 30 minutes of arrival on the unit; otherwise, return the blood to the blood bank. Blood may not be stored in the unit refrigerator.
- Stay with the patient for the first 15 minutes of the infusion. Monitor closely for signs of complications.
- Complications that may occur during infusion include high fever, sudden chills, headache, flushing, tachycardia, hypotension, itching, hives, rash, wheezing, shortness of breath, lower back pain, distention of neck veins, oppressive feeling in chest, and sense of impending doom. Should any of these symptoms occur, stop the infusion, start saline to run slowly, stay with the patient, and notify another nurse to call the physician. (The student also should notify the instructor.)
- Vital signs are taken after 15 minutes and then every half hour until the infusion is complete.
- **Do not allow blood to hang for more than 4 hours.**
- If a reaction occurs, return the unit of blood to the blood bank with the appropriate information concerning the reaction.
- Monitor the patient closely for an additional hour after the transfusion. Continue to monitor during the following days for delayed reactions such as hematuria (blood in the urine).

Principles for Administration of Total Parenteral Nutrition

- Placement of a central venous catheter must be verified by x-ray before the infusion of the total parenteral nutrition (TPN) solution is begun, unless the catheter was placed using fluoroscopy.
- Use an infusion pump to administer the TPN solution; start infusion slowly at first and then increase to the desired rate over a 24-hour period.
- Check the amount actually infusing every 30 to 60 minutes; do not rely solely on the pump functioning accurately.
- Monitor the patient's blood glucose every 4 to 6 hours per orders. Administer sliding-scale insulin as ordered for elevated blood glucose readings.
- Monitor continually for signs of complications such as glucose intolerance, infection, fluid volume excess, phlebitis, and sepsis.
- Record the intake and output accurately.
- Never speed up the solution flow rate beyond that ordered, even if it falls behind for some reason.
- The TPN infusion must be tapered before being discontinued to prevent hypoglycemia.

■ PERIOPERATIVE CARE

Preparing the Preoperative Patient for Surgery

- Check that the surgical consent has been signed.
- Check whether a blood permit was required and, if so, that it was signed.

- Verify that the complete blood count, urinalysis, and other required diagnostic test data are on the chart.
- Have the patient bathe or shower and dress in a clean gown only (no underwear).
- Check that the preoperative medications are available on the unit.
- Send the preoperative medication with the patient to the OR.
- Remove jewelry, and place all valuables in an envelope for safekeeping or give them to a family member. (A wedding band may be tied or taped in place.)
- Check and inquire about any piercings with body jewelry on any place on the body. If metal jewelry is left in place, the patient may be burned by the electrical cautery used during surgery. Remove the jewelry and secure it according to agency policy.
- Remove all metal pins from hair.
- Prepare the preoperative checklist form that accompanies the patient to surgery.
- One-half hour before the patient is expected to go to surgery, have him or her empty the bladder and remove dentures (if required).
- Prepare and administer any ordered preoperative medication at the time it is scheduled to be taken, with the supervision of the instructor or nurse as required.
- Lower the bed, raise the side rails if sedation was given, place the call light within reach, and caution the patient not to get up.
- Finish charting in nurse's notes.
- The area to be operated on (for example, the right knee) is marked with indelible ink before the surgical procedure with the patient's verification, either in the patient's room or in the holding room in the surgical suite; follow agency protocol. This is best done before preoperative medication is administered.
- When the transporter comes to take the patient to surgery, the patient is correlated with the transport slip, using two patient identifiers on the chart and patient ID band. Usually the name and hospital ID number are used. Correlate the procedure and site with the chart and the patient. The chart and the patient are correlated in the same manner.

Safety Guidelines for Surgery

The Joint Commission has issued guidelines for preventing wrong site, wrong procedure, and wrong person surgery. The nurses on regular hospital units implement the following actions, which are part of a universal protocol.

PREOPERATIVE VERIFICATION PROCESS

Verification of the correct person, procedure, and site should occur with the patient involved, awake, and aware, if possible:

- At the time of admission to the unit.
- Whenever care of the patient is transferred to another.
- Before the patient leaves the unit to enter the procedure or surgical suite.

MARKING THE OPERATIVE SITE

A mark with a sufficiently permanent marker is placed at or near the incision site that will be visible after the patient's skin is prepared and draped. (Marking is exempted for single-organ surgery, cardiac catheterization, and tooth surgery, and on premature infants, on whom the marker may leave a permanent tattoo.) Preparation should not remove the mark. The marking is done by the person performing the procedure or surgery. Marking of the correct site should be performed before the patient leaves for the procedure room or surgical suite.

DIAGNOSTIC TEST RESULTS ON HAND

Any x-rays, computed tomography (CT) scans, or magnetic resonance imaging (MRI) of the area to be involved in the procedure or surgery must be on hand in the procedure or surgical suite before the patient's arrival.

"TIME-OUT" IMMEDIATELY BEFORE THE PROCEDURE IS STARTED

Before the procedure is begun, a time-out is called, wherein all members of the surgical or procedure team check the record, operative permit, and site marked; question the patient; and view any x-ray, CT, or MRI records to ascertain that the correct site is indeed marked. The procedure or surgery is not started until all questions or concerns are resolved. The unit nurse explains this protocol to the patient so that he or she will know what to expect.

Care and Assessment of the Postoperative Patient on Return to the Clinical Unit

- Obtain the report from the recovery room nurse who cared for the patient in the postanesthesia care unit (PACU).
- Note the time of return to the unit; quickly scan the postoperative orders.
- Transfer the patient to the bed and provide warmth.
- Take vital signs; compare them with previous data.
- Assess the wound and dressing; check drains; note amount and type of drainage; check or connect/compress wound suction devices.
- Position the patient for safety and comfort (usually on the side with the head up 15 to 30 degrees). Raise side rails per agency protocol until patient is fully alert.
- Assess color and temperature of the skin.
- Assess area/system involved in the procedure (e.g., check abdominal girth, distal pulses, movement of body parts).
- Check length of each tube for patency and function: urinary catheter, IV lines, chest tubes, and oxygen cannula. Attach tube to drainage device or suction as ordered.
- Check IV infusion for correct solution, additives, and rate of flow; assess site.
- Assess urinary status: time of last voiding, amount of fluids infused, bladder distention, urge to void, and amount of hourly output via catheter. (**Do not infuse IV fluid containing potassium until urine output is at least 30 mL/hr.**)
- Assess neurological status: level of consciousness, orientation, ease of arousal, and ability to move extremities.
- Assess pain: verbal complaints, body language and time of previous analgesia, if any; medicate as needed per orders.
- Assess for nausea; medicate as needed per orders.
- Attach call light, and place emesis basin and tissues within reach.
- Assure the patient that the surgery is over and that he or she is safely back in the nursing unit.
- Allow family members to see the patient briefly.

Guidelines for Traction, Pin, or Fixator Care

- Check the physician's order regarding the type of traction and amount of weight to be used.
- Assess the traction setup and verify that:
  - Weights are hanging free.
  - Patient's body is in correct alignment.
  - Traction components are positioned and functioning properly.
- **Assess for adequate circulation and sensation; check skin temperature.**
- Perform pin care as ordered if pins are in place.
- Do not use the fixator parts as leverage for moving the patient or a limb.
- Make the bed with an assistant from top to bottom, rather than side to side.
- Keep linens smooth under the patient.
- Obtain a trapeze bar so that the patient can assist with repositioning.
- Assess the area of injury for signs of infection; check for "hot" areas, drainage, and foul smell.
- Assess the need for pain medication on a regular schedule.
- Assess for systemic signs of infection (e.g., elevated white blood cell count, elevated temperature, increasing malaise).
- Offer bedpan frequently or on a set schedule per patient's elimination pattern.
- Track frequency of bowel movements, and take action if none occur for 3 days.
- Supervise range-of-motion exercises for other joints, especially in older patients.

Postoperative Exercises to Prevent Complications

- Place the patient in a sitting position, preferably on the side of the bed so that lung expansion is not restricted by the mattress. Semi-Fowler's or side position with the head of the bed elevated 30 to 40 degrees may be used.
- If the patient has a thoracic or an abdominal incision, splint the area with a small pillow or tightly folded towel; show the patient how to do this. Hold the splinting material tightly over the incision.
- Ask the patient to inhale as deeply as possible through the nose, hold the breath for a count of five, and then slowly exhale completely through the mouth; repeat four to six times.
- On the last deep breath, ask the patient to cough forcibly on exhalation. If he or she is unable to perform a full cough, ask the patient to exhale forcibly with the mouth open several times in a row to "huff" cough and move secretions up the bronchial tree so that they can be expectorated.
- Repeat deep breathing and coughing at least every 2 hours, and ask the patient to deep breathe every hour, or whenever a commercial comes on the TV or a page of reading material is turned. **This is the most effective way to prevent postoperative respiratory complications.**

USING THE INCENTIVE SPIROMETER CORRECTLY
Teach the patient to do the following:
- Place the mouthpiece in the mouth, and completely cover it with the lips.
- Take a slow, deep breath and hold it for at least 3 seconds.

- Remove the mouthpiece and exhale slowly, with the lips puckered.
- Breathe normally for a few breaths.
- Increase the inspired volume, if possible, by 100 mL with each breath.
- When maximal volume is attained, attempt to reach it 10 times, resting a few breaths in between each attempt.

LEG EXERCISES

- Ask the patient to flex each foot firmly, pointing the toes toward the ceiling, and then to extend the foot fully and firmly. This action contracts and relaxes the calf and thigh muscles (gastrocnemius and quadriceps). Repeat five times.
- Ask the patient to rotate the ankles so that the toes draw circles, first in one direction and then the other. Repeat five times.
- Ask the patient to raise and lower the legs by bending and flexing at the knee; repeat five times. If the patient has an abdominal incision, raise the head of the bed 30 to 40 degrees before doing this exercise to relieve pressure on the abdominal muscles.
- Ask the patient to press the back of the knee against the mattress and then relax it if quadriceps-setting exercises are ordered. Repeat 10 to 12 times an hour.

TURNING IN BED AND AMBULATION

- Assist the patient to turn in bed at least every 2 hours (preferably every hour) in a side-to-back-to-side pattern as permitted. Position the patient in proper body alignment, providing pillow support to the back, leg joints, and arms as needed.
- Prepare the patient by having him or her turn to the side and then push up to a sitting position, or raise the head of the bed with the patient supine and then pivot the legs and upper body so that he or she is sitting on the side of the bed.
- Allow the patient to sit on the side of the bed with the feet supported either on the floor or on a stool. (Place slippers on the feet.) Allow several minutes of sitting the first time up after surgery. Otherwise, a couple of minutes should be sufficient before the patient rises to a standing position.
- Assist the patient to a standing position, and allow time for stabilization of blood pressure before beginning ambulation. Support the patient appropriately.
- Assist with ambulation by providing the needed amount of support and assistance. Have the patient ambulate half the total distance planned because he or she will need to return to the bed or chair.
- Rubber-soled slippers are safest for ambulation. Provide warmth with a robe or other cover as needed. Remember to remove the robe before placing the patient back on the bed.

Postoperative Hip Replacement Assessment

BASIC ASSESSMENT

- Assess pain (e.g., related to surgery or chronic pain of degenerative joint disease).
- Assess blood drainage and wound site (e.g., drain at the surgical site with a suction device).

- Check position to prevent dislocation of the prosthesis (e.g., narrower end of abduction wedge is secured between the thighs if one is ordered; when seated, the hips are not flexed beyond a 90-degree angle).
- Assess for signs of deep vein thrombosis (DVT) (e.g., Homans' sign, pain, swelling).

LAB VALUES TO CHECK
- Hematocrit and hemoglobin
- Electrolytes
- Prothrombin time, INR, or activated partial prothrombin time (aPPT)

NURSING DIAGNOSES AND INTERVENTIONS
- Acute pain:
  - Assess for pain and encourage patient to report pain when it begins.
  - Reinforce instructions on patient-controlled analgesia (PCA).
  - Provide comfort measures: keep linens smooth and clean.
- Impaired physical mobility:
  - Reposition q2h or PRN.
  - Encourage range-of-motion (ROM) and exercises to improve muscle strength and joint flexibility.
  - Teach use of walker.
- Deficient knowledge:
  - Explain that the patient should perform no flexion of the hip past 90 degrees, no internal rotation, and no adduction of the affected leg.
  - Advise to report pain in hip, buttock, or thigh, or continued limp.

■ WHAT TO DO BEFORE YOU CALL THE PHYSICIAN

Be prepared to tell the physician and use the SBAR format (Situation, Background, Assessment, Recommendation). Incorporate the following information:

1. Who you are and where you are calling from
2. What happened:
   a. Relevant background information
   b. What you tried
   c. What you want
   d. If possible, prepare and organize other questions about less urgent matters to avoid another call:
      i. Take a full, current set of vital signs (e.g., several minutes before calling physician).
      ii. Obtain pulse oximeter reading and blood glucose value if patient has change of mental status.
      iii. Carefully assess patient so that you can fully describe the problem; have current lab results, vital signs, and the medication administration record (MAR) in hand.
      iv. Consult with charge nurse if you are unsure about urgency versus waiting (e.g., it's 3:00 AM; can this matter wait until the physician arrives for AM rounds?).
      v. Be prepared to report the baseline and any changes (e.g., usually alert and conversant is now lethargic with slurred speech).

      vi. Seek an apparent cause for concern before calling (e.g., Foley not draining because tube is kinked).

     vii. Try to resolve problem if possible (e.g., use position change or distraction for pain).

    viii. Have chart with pertinent lab values in front of you before you dial.

      ix. Have a blank sheet of paper available to jot notes and orders.

■ PERINATAL CARE

Postpartum Assessment Guide

- Vital signs
- Breasts: engorgement, nipple condition, areas of warmth, redness, breastfeeding
- Uterus: fundus position, firmness
- Bowels: bowel sounds, bowel movement
- Bladder: distention, voiding
- Lochia: amount, color, clots, odor
- Episiotomy: appearance, edema, bruising, redness, drainage, approximation
- Perineum: presence of hemorrhoids—size, appearance
- C-section incision (if present): approximation, drainage, redness, tenderness
- Extremities: signs of thrombophlebitis, ability to ambulate
- Pain: location, character, severity, use of relief measures, need for analgesia
- Emotional status: family interaction, signs of depression
- Attachment: interest in newborn, eye contact, touch contact, ability to respond to infant cries

Assisting the New Mother to Breastfeed

- Have the mother wash her hands before beginning.
- Position the mother comfortably sitting with back and arm supported, supporting infant with cradle hold or football hold and pillows for proper height to breast **or** in a side-lying position with pillow beneath head, arm above head, and supporting infant in side-lying position at breast level.
- Have her turn infant's body to face her.
- Instruct her to stroke infant's face with the nipple at the lower lip.
- Have her use a "C" position to hold the breast with the thumb above the nipple and the fingers below it; the nipple should not point upward.
- As infant opens the mouth, have mother insert the nipple and areola into the mouth.
- If breast tissue blocks the infant's nose, have mother lift the infant slightly.
- Instruct mother to nurse the infant for at least 10 minutes before changing to the other breast; if infant is sucking vigorously, she should continue on this breast.
- Instruct mother to break suction by placing a finger in the corner of infant's mouth or indenting breast tissue at the mouth.
- Change position of the infant to nurse on the other breast.
- Have mother place a safety pin on the strap for the opposite breast from where nursing began this session so she knows to start on the other breast next time.
- Instruct mother to nurse at least every 3 hours initially. Exposing the nipples for 10 minutes to air and sunshine helps prevent or heal soreness.

Estimation of Lochia Volume

Scant: Less than a 2-inch (5-cm) stain on perineal pad
Light: Less than a 4-inch (10-cm) stain on perineal pad
Moderate: Less than a 6-inch (15-cm) stain on perineal pad
Large or heavy: More than a 6-inch (15-cm) stain on perineal pad, or 1 pad saturated within 2 hours
Excessive: Saturation of a perineal pad within 15 minutes (report immediately)

From Leifer G: *Introduction to maternity & pediatric nursing,* ed 6, Philadelphia, 2011, Saunders.

Fundus Massage

When the postpartum uterus is boggy or soft and is felt higher than the umbilicus, institute massage to encourage contraction. Check for bladder distention; if it is distended, have the mother void or catheterize her as needed before this procedure.

- With the woman in a supine position with the knees slightly flexed, lower the perineal pad so that you can observe the lochia as you massage the fundus.
- Place the outer edge of your nondominant hand just above the symphysis pubis and press downward slightly to anchor the lower portion of the uterus.
- Locate and massage the uterine fundus with the flat portion of the fingers of your dominant hand in a firm, circular motion.
- When the fundus is firm, keep the lower hand in place and gently push downward toward the vaginal outlet with the upper hand to expel blood and clots that have accumulated inside the uterus.
- Document the procedure and the result; note the amount of blood and clots expelled.

Apgar Scoring

Sign	0	1	2
Heart rate	Absent	Below 100 bpm	100 bpm or higher
Respiratory effort	No spontaneous respirations	Slow; weak cry	Spontaneous, with a strong, lusty cry
Muscle tone	Limp	Minimal flexion of extremities; sluggish movement	Active spontaneous motion; flexed body posture
Reflex irritability	No response to suction or gentle slap on soles	Minimal response (grimace) to stimulation	Prompt response to suction and to gentle slap on sole of foot
Color	Blue or pale	Body pink, extremities blue	Completely pink (light skin) or absence of cyanosis (dark skin)

A score of 8-10 requires just continued observation and support of adaptation; a score of 4-7 means the infant needs gentle stimulation such as rubbing the back; a score of 3 or lower means that the infant needs immediate active resuscitation.
Adapted from Leifer G: *Introduction to maternity & pediatric nursing,* ed 7, St Louis, 2015, Saunders.

Clinical Quick Reference

Umbilical Cord Care

The following procedure is to be done with each diaper change per facility protocol:

- Check clamp for tight closure.
- Assess for presence of three vessels unless dried.
- Lift the cord gently away from the abdomen for ease of cleaning all areas.
- Let the cord dry naturally, and keep it above the top of the diaper.
- Observe cord and abdominal attachment area for redness, discharge, or foul odor.
- Document observations and care.

■ GUIDELINES FOR ATTENDING CLINICAL IN A PSYCHIATRIC FACILITY

Dress: Street clothes, no lab coat or uniform. Avoid clothes with pictures or printing that could stimulate delusional thinking in the wrong direction by patients. Avoid tightly fitted clothes that are too revealing and sexually suggestive. Limit jewelry to stud earrings without dangles or hoops. No neck attire of any sort. Shoes must be low-heeled with closed toe area. Wear name pin for identification at all times.

Grooming: Hair should be pulled back and confined so that it cannot be grabbed easily.

Safety: Be alert to sudden sounds such as banging, loud voices, change of lighting, and new/strange smells. If these are encountered, turn toward that disturbance to assess the situation, and back up toward a safer area if need is indicated.

Symptoms of Post-Traumatic Stress Disorder (PTSD)

PTSD can cause many symptoms, but watch for these:

- Re-experiencing symptoms
  - Flashbacks: reliving the trauma over and over, including physical symptoms
  - Bad dreams
  - Frightening thoughts
- Avoidance symptoms
  - Staying away from places events, or objects that are reminders of the experience
  - Feeling emotionally numb
  - Feeling strong guilt, depression, or worry
  - Losing interest in activities that were enjoyable in the past
  - Having trouble remembering the dangerous event
- Hyperarousal symptoms
  - Being easily startled
  - Feeling tense of "on edge"
  - Having difficulty sleeping and/or having angry outbursts

From Post-Traumatic Stress Disorder (PTSD), http://www.nimh.nih.gov/health/publications/post-traumatic-stress-disorder-ptsd/index.shtml.

■ CARING FOR A PATIENT WITH ALZHEIMER'S OR OTHER DEMENTIA

- Allow extra time for accomplishing activities of daily living.
- Limit the number of choices you give.
- When the patient becomes agitated, use a distraction such as food, drink, music, or conversation.
- Match what you say with a corresponding action.
- Maintain eye contact and a comfortable posture.
- Identify what is triggering an undesirable behavior, and modify the environment.
- Label common items with pictures and or words (e.g., toilet for bathroom door, lightbulb at the light switch, clothes on the closet door).
- Keep room well lit at all times without causing shadows.
- Involve patient in activities that require use of large muscle groups.
- Give the patient something to do or hold while you assist with carrying out a task (e.g., hold the toothpaste, an item of clothing, a washcloth).
- Approach the patient with a calm manner, smile, and gentle tone of voice.
- Use simple words and short sentences, and explain why you are there and what you are going to do. Use a picture flash card to help orient the patient to the task.
- Do not take combativeness or reluctance to do something personally; it is the disease causing the problem, not the patient.
- When the patient is resistant to doing something, try to figure out what he or she is feeling and express that to the patient. Sometimes this approach helps with cooperation.

Clinical Quick Reference

■ NUTRITION

Rehydration Formula for Dehydration from Vomiting and Diarrhea

Mix together:

2 quarts water
1 tsp. baking soda
1 tsp. salt
7 T. sugar
A packet of sugar-free Kool-Aid or other sugar-free drink mix may be added. Can be frozen into ice cubes or into ice pops.

Alternative Seasoning Mix (*Makes* ¼ *Cup*)

1 T. dry mustard   5 tsp. onion powder
1 tsp. thyme   1 T. garlic powder
½ tsp. white pepper   1 T. paprika
½ tsp. celery seed

Store in a closed container.

A Guide to Daily Food Choices

Use MyPlate (Figure 5-8) from the U.S. Department of Agriculture (USDA) to help people eat better every day. General recommendations from the USDA (2011) for the general population include the following:

- Enjoying food but eating less of it
- Avoiding oversized portions
- Increasing intake of fruits, vegetables, and whole grains
- Choosing low-fat or fat-free dairy products
- Reducing intake of sodium
- Drinking water instead of sugary beverages
- Making physical activity an everyday occurrence
- Additional tips and resources, including recipes and interactive tools, are available at choosemyplate.gov.

Note the specific Dietary Guidelines from the USDA:

- **Fruits and vegetables:** Consume 2 cups of fruit and $2\frac{1}{2}$ cups of vegetables daily. Make fruits and vegetables half of what is eaten at each meal. Choose fiber-rich fruits and vegetables.
- **Whole grains:** Consume 6 ounces daily. Eat three 1-ounce portions of whole grains. Choose whole, unsweetened grains when possible.
- **Dairy products:** Drink 3 cups of skim or low-fat milk, or eat the equivalent dairy products (e.g., low-fat yogurt, low-fat cheese).
- **Protein:** Eat $5\frac{1}{2}$ ounces of poultry, lean meat, fish, beans, or nuts. Eat meat rarely. Choose lean meats and poultry. Bake, broil, or grill meat, poultry, and fish choices.

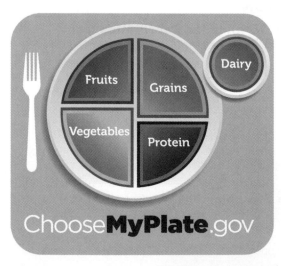

FIGURE 5-8 MyPlate. (From U.S. Department of Health and Human Services/U.S. Department of Agriculture, 2011. www.choosemyplate.gov.)

- **Oils and sweets:** Consume 6 teaspoons per day, used sparingly. Use healthful oils such as olive, canola, and safflower. Sugar should be limited. Keep total fat intake between 20% and 35% of calories, with most fats coming from sources of polyunsaturated and monounsaturated fatty acids, such as fish, nuts, and vegetable oils. Consume less than 7% of calories from saturated fatty acids and less than 300 mg/day of cholesterol, and keep *trans* fatty acid consumption as low as possible.
- Calorie control is to be considered as well for a healthy diet. Combine a healthy diet with sufficient exercise to maintain a healthy weight.

Choice Equivalents within Each Food Group

Servings based on a 2000-calorie diet:

- **Fruits:** 2 cups of fruit a day. Eat a variety and use fresh, frozen, canned, or dried fruit rather than fruit juice. A serving could be 1 small banana, 1 medium orange, or $\frac{1}{4}$ cup of dried apricots or peaches.
- **Vegetables:** $2\frac{1}{2}$ cups a day. In particular, select from all five vegetable subgroups (dark green, orange, legumes, starchy vegetables, and other vegetables) several times a week. Eat portions of vegetables for lunch and dinner.
- **Grains:** 6 ounces per day; 3-ounce equivalents a day of whole-grain products. Half the grains should be whole grains. One ounce is 1 slice of bread, 1 cup of breakfast cereal, or $\frac{1}{2}$ cup of cooked rice or pasta.
- **Protein:** $5\frac{1}{2}$ ounces of poultry, lean meat, fish, beans, or nuts per day. Equivalent servings of 1 ounce of meat, fish, or poultry are as follows: 1 egg, $\frac{1}{4}$ cup cooked beans, 1 tablespoon peanut butter, $\frac{1}{2}$ ounce of nuts or seeds, and $\frac{1}{4}$ cup tofu. A 4-ounce serving of meat, fish, or poultry for dinner should be about the size of a normal deck of cards or the palm of the hand. Eat two 4-ounce servings of fish per week. Choose a variety of protein foods.
- **Dairy products:** 3 cups of milk per day; 1 cup of milk equals 8 ounces. Equivalent servings to 1 cup of milk are 1 cup of low-fat or nonfat yogurt, $\frac{1}{2}$ ounce of low-fat cheese such as Swiss, Gouda, Roquefort, and white string cheese. Two ounces of low-fat or fat-free processed cheese such as American or Laughing Cow is equal to 1 cup of milk.
- **Fats:** 6 teaspoons per day. One teaspoon of liquid oil is equal to 1 teaspoon of tub margarine, 1 tablespoon of mayonnaise, or 2 teaspoons of light salad dressing.

Key Recommendations

ALL POPULATIONS

- Engage in regular physical activity, and reduce sedentary activities to promote health, psychological well-being, and a healthy body weight.
- Balance body weight in a healthy range; balance calories from foods and beverages with calories expended. Eat a more plant-based diet.
- Those who choose to drink alcoholic beverages should do so sensibly and in moderation—defined as the consumption of up to one drink per day for women and up to two drinks per day for men.
- Consume less than 1 gm of sodium (approximately 1 tsp of salt) per day. Choose and prepare foods with little salt. At the same time, consume

potassium-rich foods, such as fruits and vegetables. Age 51 and older: limit sodium to 1500 mg per day.

CHILDREN AND ADOLESCENTS

Children 2 to 8 years of age should consume 2 cups per day of fat-free or low-fat milk or equivalent milk products. Children 9 years of age and older should consume 3 cups per day of fat-free or low-fat milk or equivalent milk products.

WOMEN OF CHILDBEARING AGE WHO MAY BECOME PREGNANT

Eat iron-rich plant foods or iron-fortified foods along with vitamin C–rich foods. Consume adequate folate foods daily or adequate synthetic folic acid from a supplement.

WOMEN IN THE FIRST TRIMESTER OF PREGNANCY

Consume adequate synthetic folic acid daily from fortified foods or supplements in addition to folate food forms.

PEOPLE OLDER THAN 50 YEARS OF AGE

- Consume vitamin B_{12} in its crystalline form (i.e., fortified foods or supplements).
- Older adults, people with dark skin, and people exposed to insufficient ultraviolet sunlight: consume extra vitamin D from vitamin D–fortified foods and/or supplements.

Body Mass Index

The body mass index (BMI) is based on the relationship of weight to height. It is independent of body frame size. BMI is used to determine whether a person has excess fat. Body mass is calculated with the following formula:

$$BMI = \frac{Weight\ (lb)}{Height\ (in)^2} \times 705$$

In the adult, a score of 20 to 25 is within normal and is associated with the least risk of early death.

Example: A woman 5 feet 4 inches tall, weighing 122 pounds:

$$Height\ squared = 64\ in \times 64\ in = 4096$$
$$122 \div 4096 = 0.0297085$$
$$0.029785 \times 705 = 20.9$$

This woman's body mass index is 20.9.

Therapeutic Diets

CLEAR LIQUID DIET

Purpose. Provides an oral source of calories and electrolytes as a means of preventing dehydration and reducing colonic residue to a minimum.

Indications. The immediate postoperative period, acute debilitation, acute gastroenteritis, upper gastrointestinal lesions; also to reduce the amount of residue in the colon in preparation for bowel surgery, barium enema, or after colon surgery.

Type of Food	Foods Included	Foods Excluded
Beverage	Carbonated beverages, tea, coffee, strained fruit juice (apple, cranberry, cran-apple, grape, punch, powdered fruit beverage mixes, electrolyte replacement drinks)	Milk, milk drinks
Soup	Fat-free bouillon or broth, consommé	Any other
Dessert	Plain gelatin, Popsicles, fruit ice	Any other
Condiments	Sugar, honey, plain hard candy	Any other, caffeine, artificial sweetener

FULL LIQUID DIET

Indications. Oral surgery, mandibular fracture, plastic surgery to the face, esophageal strictures; also for acutely ill patients for whom chewing may be difficult, or other postoperative states in transition between a clear liquid and another diet; three to six small feedings a day are recommended.

Contraindications. Nausea, vomiting, distention, or diarrhea when advanced to this diet postoperatively; lactose intolerance.

Type of Food	Foods Included	Foods Excluded
Beverage	Carbonated beverages, coffee, tea, fruit juices, milk, milk drinks, vegetable juices (strained), eggnog	None
Bread	None	All
Cereal	Soft-cooked cereals (gruels)	Any other
Fat	Butter, cream, margarine	Any other
Vegetables	Tomato juice, vegetable puree in soup	Any other
Meat, egg, cheese	Raw pasteurized eggs*; soft-cooked egg sometimes allowed	Any other
Soup	Broth, strained cream soups, yogurt	Any other
Dessert	Yogurt, custard, ice cream (plain), pudding, tapioca, sherbets, plain gelatin	Any other
Condiments	Pepper, salt, cinnamon, nutmeg, sugar, honey, hard candy, syrup, pureed meat and vegetables for soup only	Any other

*Raw, unpasteurized eggs should not be used because of the danger of *Salmonella* infection. In addition, the avidin in the egg white prevents the absorption of biotin.

Adapted from Peckenpaugh N, Poleman C: *Nutrition essentials and diet therapy*, ed 11, Philadelphia, 2010, Saunders.

SOFT, LOW-FIBER (BLAND) DIET

Indications. Gastrointestinal disturbances, general physical weakness, or poor chewing ability.

Note. Soft diet contains whole pieces of food that are not chopped or pureed. Some elements of this soft diet may have to be adjusted in consistency to fit the needs of a particular patient (e.g., pureed meats, fruits).

Type of Food	Foods Included	Foods Excluded
Beverage	Carbonated beverages, decaffeinated coffee or tea, milk, milk drinks	Alcoholic, cocoa, or caffeinated beverages
Bread	White or fine rye bread or rolls, soda crackers, waffles, graham crackers, muffins, cornbread	Whole-grain products, any breads with nuts, seeds, or dried fruits
Cereal	Cream of wheat or rice cereals	Whole-grain cereals, bran, cereals cooked with nuts, seeds, or fruits, hard or firm dry cereal
Fats	Butter, cream, margarine, salad dressing, gravy, mayonnaise, sour cream	Fried foods
Fruit	Fruit juices, ripe avocado, banana, cooked or canned apples, apricots, cherries, pears; all of the listed fruit without skin or seeds; dried fruit puree	Raw fruits, skins, or seeds; citrus juice or fruit; pineapple; cranberries
Vegetables	Cooked, pureed vegetables; vegetable juice	Raw vegetables or skins, broccoli, cabbage, cauliflower, mild or hot peppers, sauerkraut, avocado, tomatoes or tomato products
Potato or substitute	Potatoes, sweet potatoes, rice, spaghetti, grits, macaroni, noodles	None
Meat, eggs, cheese	Ground or tender nonstringy meat, fish, or chicken; eggs; cottage cheese; cheddar or American cheese; yogurt; tofu; and smooth peanut butter	Fried meat, chicken, or fish; strong cheeses; dried cooked beans; processed spicy meats
Soup	Puree from food allowed, all cream and broth soups	Whole vegetable or meat soups unless adjusted in consistency for patient, tomato-based soup, chili
Dessert	Custard, gelatin, angel food cake, tapioca, puddings, ice cream, cake, plain cookies, hard candy	Rich desserts, nuts, raisins, coconut
Condiments	Salt, white pepper, sugar, vinegar, sauces, gravy, ketchup, honey, syrup, jelly	Olives, pickles, popcorn, relishes, black pepper, strong spices, chili

Data from Medline Plus: *Bland diet.* Updated December 2, 2011. http://www.nlm.nih.gov/medlineplus/ency/patientinstructions/000068.htm.

American Heart Association Guidelines for a Heart-Healthy Diet and Lifestyle

The American Heart Association's recommendations include the following points:

- Consume an overall healthy diet.
- Maintain a healthy body weight by balancing calories consumed with calories burned.
- Be aware of your daily caloric requirements and increase awareness of the calorie content of various food portions.
- Obtain at least 30 minutes of physical activity each day.
- Eat a variety of fruits and vegetables (not fruit juices), adding deeply colored ones such as spinach, carrots, peaches, and berries.
- Limit carbohydrate choices to whole-grain, high-fiber foods, decreasing refined grains such as white bread and white rice.
- Consume food-based sources of fiber (legumes, whole-grains, fruits, and vegetables).
- No more than half of discretionary calories should come from added sugars.
- Have two servings of fish relatively high in omega-3 fatty acids twice a week. (Pregnant women and children should avoid mercury-contaminated fish.)
- Choose extra-lean meats and low-fat (<5 g total fat) or fat-free dairy products; limit intake of saturated fat, *trans* fat, and cholesterol.
- Use non–animal-based sources of protein such as legumes and beans.
- Consume less than 10% of calories from saturated fats. Keep *trans* fat consumption to no more than 3 g per day (based on a 2000-calorie diet).
- Take in few beverages and foods with added sugars, including high-fructose corn syrup.
- Keep sodium consumption down to 2300 mg daily; prepare foods with little or no salt. Middle-age and older adults, African-Americans, and those with hypertension should limit sodium intake to 1500 mg of sodium per day.
- Limit alcohol to one drink per day for women and two drinks per day for men (1 drink = 12 oz of beer, 4 oz of wine, 1.5 oz of 80-proof distilled spirits, or 1 oz of 100-proof spirits).
- Take in vitamins A, C, D, E, and B_{12} through vitamin-rich foods and/or supplements.
- At all times be aware of portion size; when eating out, select vegetables and fruits, and avoid foods prepared with added saturated or *trans* fat, salt, and sugar.

Data from American Heart Association: Diet and lifestyle recommendations. Updated May 21, 2010. http://www.heart.org/HEARTORG/GettingHealthy/NutritionCenter/HealthyEating/The-American-Heart-Associations-Diet-and-Lifestyle-Recommendations_UCM_305855_Article.jsp.

Clinical Quick Reference

Low-Fat Diet

Frequently Consumed High-Fat Foods	Alternative Foods
Fried foods	Roast, bake, grill, stir-fry, or broil foods when possible.
	Baste meats with broth or stock.
	Use nonstick cookware and an aerosol cooking spray.
Fatty meats (bacon, sausage, choice grade meats, poultry, frankfurters, luncheon meats)	Choose two or three servings of meat and shellfish or fish with a daily total of about 6 oz.
	Choose a vegetarian entrée (dried beans, peas) at least once a week.
	Trim visible fat from meat; remove skin from poultry before eating.
	Choose beef grade "select," which contains less fat marbling; leaner cuts of meat include flank, sirloin, or tenderloin; loin pork chops.
	Marinate lean cuts of meat in lemon juice, flavored vinegars, or fruit juices.
Cheese (aged and cream cheeses)	Choose cheese with 6 g or less of fat per ounce such as farmer's cheese.
High-fat snacks (chips, some crackers, dips)	Substitute with pretzels, low-fat crackers, air-popped popcorn.
Salad dressing, mayonnaise, sour cream	Use fat-free or reduced-fat salad dressings and sour cream.
	Substitute plain low-fat yogurt for mayonnaise or sour cream.
	Rely on mustard and salad greens to add moisture to sandwiches rather than high-fat spreads.
Gravies	Use the paste method for making gravy or sauces (add flour or cornstarch to cold liquids slowly and blend well).
Homogenized whole milk products	Use skim milk, buttermilk, low-fat yogurt, and cottage cheese.
Margarine and seasonings such as lard, bacon, and ham	Use jam, jelly, or marmalade spread instead of butter or margarine.
	Season with herbs, lemon juice, or stock rather than lard, bacon, or ham.
Breads and cereals	Plain bread, rolls, graham crackers, matzoh, saltines, pretzels, most cereals.

DASH (Dietary Approaches to Stop Hypertension) Eating Plan

Research has shown that the DASH combination eating plan lowers blood pressure and therefore may help prevent and control high blood pressure. This diet is rich in fruits, vegetables, and low-fat dairy foods, and low in saturated and total fat. It is also low in cholesterol; high in dietary fiber, potassium, calcium, and magnesium; and moderately high in protein. The following DASH eating plan on is based on 2000 calories a day. Depending on caloric needs, the number of daily servings in a food group may vary from those listed.

DASH (Dietary Approaches to Stop Hypertension) Eating Plan (cont'd)

Food Group	Daily Servings	Serving Sizes	Examples and Notes	Significance of Each Food Group to the DASH Diet Pattern
Grains, grain products	7-8	1 slice bread ½ cup dry cereal ½ cup cooked rice, pasta, cereal	Whole wheat bread, English muffin, pita bread, bagel, cereals, grits, oatmeal	Major sources of energy, fiber
Vegetables	4-5	1 cup raw leafy vegetables ½ cup cooked vegetable 6 oz vegetable juice	Tomatoes, potatoes, carrots, peas, squash, broccoli, turnip greens, collards, kale, spinach, artichokes, sweet potatoes, beans	Rich sources of potassium, magnesium, fiber
Fruits	4-5	6 oz fruit juice 1 medium fruit ½ cup dried fruit ½ cup fresh, frozen, or canned fruit	Apricots, bananas, dates, oranges, orange juice, grapefruit, grapefruit juice, mangos, melons, peaches, pineapples, prunes, raisins, strawberries, tangerines	Important sources of potassium, magnesium, fiber
Low-fat, nonfat dairy foods	2-3	8 oz milk 1 cup yogurt 1.5 oz cheese	Skim or 1% milk, skim or low-fat buttermilk, nonfat or low-fat yogurt, part-skim mozzarella cheese, nonfat juice	Major sources of calcium, protein
Meats, poultry, fish	2 or less	3 oz cooked meats, poultry, fish	Select only lean; trim away visible fats; broil, roast, or boil, instead of frying; remove skin from poultry	Rich sources of protein, magnesium
Nuts, seeds, legumes	4-5 per week	1.5 oz or ⅓ cup nuts ½ oz or 2 tbsp seeds ½ cup cooked legumes	Almonds, filberts, mixed nuts, peanuts, walnuts, sunflower seeds, kidney beans, lentils	Rich sources of energy, magnesium, potassium, protein, fiber

National Heart Lung and Blood Institute: What is the DASH eating plan? Available at http://www.nhlbi.nih.gov/files/docs/public/heart/new_dash.pdf.

Sodium-Restricted Diet

Along with foods, the sodium content of medications and local water should be considered. Potent oral diuretics have lessened the need for severe limitation of sodium in the diet.

INDICATIONS

Chronic heart failure, hypertension, atherosclerosis, edema, cirrhosis of the liver, or chronic kidney disease.

Type of Diet	Sodium Per Day Allowed	Foods Excluded
No added salt	4-5 g	No salty or high-sodium processed foods; do not add salt to food at the table; use only small amounts in cooking
Mild sodium restriction	2-3 g	No added salt; no pickles, olives, bacon; restrict ham, chips, canned soups, salted nuts, smoked meats or fish, bouillon, frozen entrées, luncheon meats, processed cheese, regular peanut butter, instant cocoa or hot cereals, cooking wine, seasoning salts, soy sauce, Worcestershire sauce, meat extracts
Moderate sodium restriction	1 g	Same foods restricted as in mild sodium diet; only low-sodium products are to be used; no restriction on commercially baked products; no cheese or canned or frozen vegetables containing salt; no more than 2 cups of milk
Severe sodium restriction	500 mg	Same foods are restricted as in moderate sodium diet; only restriction is salt-free bread; no high-sodium fruits or vegetables such as celery, carrots, beets, artichokes, Swiss chard, greens, kale, spinach, white turnips, sauerkraut, hominy

High-Fiber Diet

Fiber increases fecal bulk, holds water, and binds calcium, magnesium, and other needed nutrients. The inclusion of high-fiber foods in the diet is recommended for patients on a general diet and for those with constipation. In addition, a high-fiber diet may be helpful in the treatment of diverticular disease. High-fiber foods include whole-grain breads and cereals, bran, oatmeal, wheat germ, millet, brown rice, cornmeal, legumes (dried beans), nuts, seeds, and fresh fruits, as well as vegetables with skins (e.g., apples, grapes, apricots, raw cauliflower, carrots, celery, cabbage, lettuce). Bananas, prunes, dates, figs, and rhubarb are good laxatives and high in fiber.

High-Calorie, High-Protein, High-Vitamin Diet

This diet is indicated for underweight or malnourished patients. The normal diet is supplemented with foods high in protein, vitamins, and calories. Small, frequent feedings are best (six to eight per day). The caloric value can be 25% to 50% above normal (up to 3000 calories/day), and the protein increased to 90 to 100 g/day for adults who do not have renal insufficiency.

Cheeses, sauces, cream soups, potatoes, ice cream, pudding, and milk shakes may be used liberally. Prepared nutritional supplements such as Ensure, Ensure Plus, Sustacal, Boost, or Carnation Instant Breakfast may be used at meals or between meals. Supplementary vitamins may be indicated.

Group	Number of Servings
Milk	4 or more
Meat or meat substitutes	3 or 4
Breads and cereals	4 to 8
Fruits and vegetables	4 or more

Gluten-Free Diet

Patients with celiac disease or sprue must completely avoid gluten. Those with gluten sensitivity should avoid gluten as much as possible. A gluten-free diet should not be used to promote weight loss. Some prescription drugs, vitamins, and over-the-counter drugs contain gluten. Patients should be told to consult their pharmacist.

FOODS ALLOWED
Fruits and vegetables: Fresh, frozen, and canned fruits and vegetables and their juices

Meats and protein alternatives: Fresh meat, fish and poultry, eggs, dried beans and peas, nuts and seeds, tofu. Fresh turkey without additives.

Milk products: Milk, cream, buttermilk, yogurt, plain cheese, cream cheese, cottage cheese

Grains: Breads and baked goods made from gluten-free products, pastas made from rice, beans, corn, potato, quinoa, millet, soy, wild rice, and other gluten-free grains

Cereals: Puffed corn, amaranth, buckwheat, millet, rice, rice flakes or soy, hominy grits, soy grits, cream of buckwheat, cream of rice, puffed amaranth

Rice: Brown, white, basmati, jasmine, or wild rice, rice tortillas

Corn: Tortillas

Fats and oils: Butter, margarine, vegetable oils, lard, shortening, cream

Desserts: Gluten-free cakes, cookies, pastries; many ice creams, sorbets, sherbets, Popsicles, whipped toppings, egg custards, gelatin, most hard candies, most chocolate bars

Beverages: Cocoa drinks, soft drinks, juices, non-dairy soy; rice-, potato-, and nut-based beverages; teas, coffee; distilled alcoholic beverages such as rum, gin, whiskey, vodka, wines, and pure liqueurs; gluten-free beer, ale, and lager

Sweet condiments: Honey, jams, jellies, marmalade, molasses, corn syrup, maple syrup, sugar (white, brown, and confectioner's)

Snack foods: Plain popcorn, potato chips, corn chips, nuts, soy nuts, rice cakes, corn cakes, rice crackers

Condiments: Salad dressings without gluten-based ingredients, plain pickles, relish, olives, ketchup, mustard, tomato paste, pure herbs and spices, gluten-free soy sauce, vinegars (all but malt vinegar)

Common baking ingredients: Pure cocoa, baking chocolate, chocolate chips, carob chips and powder, cream of tartar, baking soda, yeast, brewer's yeast, vanilla

Soups, sauces, and gravies: Homemade broths, gluten-free bouillon cubes, cream soups and stocks made from allowed ingredients, sauces and gravies made from allowed ingredients

FOODS TO AVOID

Barley

Rye

Oats (unless totally gluten free)

Couscous

Hydrolyzed protein

Wheat-based soy sauce

Meat extenders and vegetarian meal substitutes

Deli meats, hot dogs, sausages, imitation seafood products unless all natural

Marinades and sauces

Baked beans

Seasoned nuts

Flavored tofu

Malted milk

Cheese sauces, cheese spreads, flavored cheeses

Seasoned or flavored rice mixes, rice pilaf

Icing or frosting

Ice creams containing wheat or wheat-containing ingredients

Dried fruits

Candy bars and soft candies; licorice

Flavored teas, coffees, and herbal teas containing barley or barley malt

Undistilled alcoholic beverages, coolers

Some brands of potato chips

Seasoned popcorn

Pretzels and crackers (regular)

Soy and teriyaki sauce

Packaged dry salad dressing mixes

Many commercial salad dressings

Instant mashed potatoes

Worchestershire sauce

Malt vinegar

Hot cocoa mix

Seasoning mixes

Pre-frozen French fries (dusted with flour)

Commercially produced soups and broths (contain wheat flour or hydrolyzed wheat protein)

Data from Case S: *Gluten-free diet: a comprehensive resource guide*, Regina, Saskatchewan, Canada, 2008, Case Nutritional Consulting Inc.

Lactose-Free Diet Foods to Avoid

Beverages: Milk, ice cream, sour cream, yogurt,* soft cheeses, mayonnaise, cream cheese, half-and-half, whipped cream, cottage cheese, evaporated milk, condensed milk, dry milk powder, breakfast drinks

Bread and pasta: Bread, biscuits, pancakes, French toast, waffles, toaster pastries, doughnuts, sweet rolls, crackers, and cakes often contain lactose from milk products

Sauces and toppings: Salad dressings containing milk or whey, cheese sauces, butter, dips, whipped toppings, sauces containing milk or milk products

Vegetables: Any au gratin, scalloped, or creamed vegetables, and vegetables with cheese sauce

Sweets: Ice cream cake, frozen yogurt, milk chocolate, puddings, custards, sherbets and desserts with sweetened condensed milk; butterscotch, caramel and toffee-flavored sweets, and some artificial sweeteners (check label)

Other food products: Many protein powders and bars, instant potatoes, soups, non-dairy liquid and powdered coffee creamers, non-dairy whipped toppings, some salad dressings, candies

---

*Yogurt with active live cultures decreases the lactose content of the product and may be tolerated.

Principles for Administering Enteral (Tube) Feedings

- Always check for proper tube placement before beginning a feeding. If feeding is continuous, check placement once per shift or before adding formula to the container.
- Elevate the head of the bed 30 to 45 degrees, and leave it up for 30 to 60 minutes after the feeding. Keep the head of the bed elevated at all times if the feeding is continuous.
- Check for gastric residual before starting the next feeding or every 4 hours. If the residual is more than half of the volume given in the last feeding, or greater than 150 mL when continuous feeding is in progress, replace the residual and delay the next feeding for 1 to 2 hours. For continuous feeding, notify the physician of the excessive residual amount.
- If nausea occurs, stop the feeding and notify the physician.
- If persistent diarrhea occurs, notify the physician.
- Monitor bowel movements.
- Check skin turgor to be certain patient is not becoming dehydrated.
- Be alert to signs of hyperglycemia during the first few days of tube feeding.
- Flush the tubing with 30 to 50 mL of water, depending on fluid requirements, after each feeding and at least once per shift.
- When giving medications, flush the tubing with 10 to 30 mL of water initially and with 10 mL of water after each medication. Do not mix medications together.
- Use elixirs rather than crushed pills whenever possible. If pills have to be crushed, crush ahead of time and mix with warm water. Never crush a sustained-release medication.
- If tubing is clogged, check with a nurse for unit protocol on unclogging tubing. Using warm water and milking the tubing is sometimes sufficient; carbonated cola is used in some facilities, and cranberry juice is used in others.

Giving Medication via Nasogastric or Small-Bore Tube

EQUIPMENT
- Clean gloves
- 50-mL barrel syringe
- Container for tap water
- pH test strip
- Stethoscope

STEPS
- Check medication with medication administration record (MAR); verify patient name, allergies.
- Perform the Six Rights of Medication Administration.
- Prepare medication (i.e., use liquid form if possible; tablets must be finely crushed and diluted in water; timed-release capsule beads should not be crushed; the beads may appear very small but will easily clog tubing; consult with instructor or staff before administering).
- Assess presence of bowel sounds, abdominal distention, nausea, or vomiting.
- Elevate head of bed (HOB) 30 to 90 degrees.
- Verify tube placement (e.g., with a 50-mL syringe, gently aspirate a few drops of stomach contents and test with pH paper). For small-bore tube, check x-ray result for correct placement and that the tube is still inserted correctly by noting where the black line is in relation to the nostril per the initial note after insertion.
- Clamp tube to prevent excess air from entering tube.
- Draw up 30 to 50 mL of water; unclamp tube and gently flush.
- Clamp tube; detach syringe and remove plunger; reattach barrel to use as funnel.
- Add liquid medication slowly and allow to instill; add water for flushing before the syringe is entirely empty to prevent excessive air from entering tube.
- Clamp tube for 30 to 60 minutes before reattaching to wall suction.
- Assess patient for nausea, fullness, and discomfort.
- Leave HOB elevated during procedure and for 30 to 60 minutes afterward.
- Clean and rinse syringe and water container; store at bedside.
- Document procedure and outcomes.

ONLINE
RESOURCES

6

Note: These listings are provided as aids for studying, class work preparation, and patient teaching. Be aware that websites come and go, and what follows are examples of online resources available for selected topics at the time of printing. The author and publisher do not endorse the websites listed.

■ RESOURCES FOR NURSING STUDENTS

ARTERIAL BLOOD GAS TUTORIAL
http://www.m2hnursing.com/ABG/basic_questions.php

ASSERTIVENESS SKILLS
http://www.michiganprosecutor.org/Downloads/Webinars/Assertiveness_Skills.pdf
http://www.ndsu.edu/counseling/self_help/assertiveness_skills/

AUSCULTATION ASSISTANT
http://www.wilkes.med.ucla.edu/intro.html

BEST PRACTICE GUIDELINES
http://www.guideline.gov/content.aspx?id=47637
http://rnao.ca/bpg/guidelines
http://rnao.ca/bpg

CARDIAC INFORMATION
www.mendedhearts.org
www.blaufuss.org/
www.med.umich.edu/lrc/psb/heartsounds/
www.easyauscultation.com/heart-sounds

CARE PLANS AND TEMPLATES
http://www.careplans.com/pages/lib/default.aspx?cid=6
http://www.rncentral.com/nursing-library/careplans
http://www.pterrywave.com/nursing/care%20plans/nursing%20care%20
    plans%20toc.aspx
http://web.nmsu.edu/~ebosman/nursing/careplan.shtml

CAREGIVER INFORMATION
www.caregiver.com
http://www.caregiversupportnetwork.com/
http://helpguide.org/home-pages/caregiving.htm

COMPLEMENTARY AND ALTERNATIVE MEDICINE

http://www.mayoclinic.org/healthy-living/consumer-health/in-depth/alternative
-medicine/art-20045267

http://nccam.nih.gov

CONCEPT MAPPING

http://ojni.org/6_2/602/strategies.htm

http://www.ehow.com/how_5526833_make-nursing-concept-map.html

http://www.slideshare.net/nytenurse/concept-mapping-100669

CULTURAL INFORMATION

http://babelfish.com (for translation)

http://depts.washington.edu/pfes/CultureClues.htm

http://health.utah.gov/disparities/culture.html

http://www.ccah-alliance.org/icetoolkit.html

DETERMINING YOUR LEARNING STYLE

http://www.ldpride.net/learning-style-test.html

http://search.usf.edu/search?q=learning+styles&x=0&y=0&client=tampa&proxy
stylesheet=usf-edu-cms&site=tampa&output=xml_no_dtd&numgm=5

DISABILITIES

www.aucd.org/

www.exceptionalnurse.com

www.washington.edu/doit/Careers/print.html?ID=314

DISTANCE LEARNING AND DEGREE PROGRAMS

http://www.elearners.com/online-degrees/nursing/

http://www.nursingdegrees.com/

www.rncentral.com

DRUG CALCULATION HELP

www.dosagehelp.com

http://www.nursesaregreat.com/drug-calculations.php

www.testandcalc.com/quiz/index.asp

ECG INFORMATION

http://cal.vet.upenn.edu/projects/lgcardiac/ecg_tutorial/introduction.htm

www.gwc.maricopa.edu/class/bio202/cyberheart/ekgqzr.htm

http://library.med.utah.edu/kw/ecg

EVIDENCE-BASED NURSING

www.ahrq.gov/clinic/cpgsix.htm

www.guideline.gov

http://hsl.mcmaster.ca/resources/topic/eb/nurse.html

http://www.cochrane.org/cochrane-reviews

FLASHCARD PROGRAMS

http://www.cram.com/tag/nursing

http://quizlet.com/

http://www.studystack.com/Nursing

FORUMS AND NETWORKING

http://onlinelpntorn.org/2011/40-best-forums-for-nursing-students/
http://allnurses.com/nursing-student
http://www.nursetogether.com/

GENERAL MEDICAL INFORMATION

http://emedicine.medscape.com/
www.healthcentral.com
http://health.nih.gov
http://www.mayoclinic.org/patient-care-and-health-information
http://ods.od.nih.gov/Health_Information/How_To_Evaluate_Health
    _Information_on_the_Internet_Questions_and_Answers.aspx
www.medscape.com
www.nlm.nih.gov/medlineplus

GENERAL NURSING RESOURCES

www.healthfinder.gov
http://www.practicalnursing.org/

GENERAL REFERENCES

www.bartleby.com
http://www.medicinenet.com/medterms-medical-dictionary/article.htm
www.merriam-webster.com
http://medical-dictionary.thefreedictionary.com/

GRANTS AND SCHOLARSHIPS

www.collegescholarships.org/grants/nursing.htm
http://edu.fastweb.com/v/o registration/flow/step1?ref=google_nursing-1f
www.oshpd.ca.gov/HPEF
www.hrsa.gov/loanscholarships/scholarships/Nursing
http://minoritynurse.com/scholarships/

NATIONAL COUNCIL LICENSURE EXAMINATION (NCLEX) INFORMATION AND STUDY TIPS

www.nclexinfo.com
www.ncsbn.org/nclex.htm
www.ncsbn.org/1268.htm
http://www.kaptest.com/NCLEX/Home/decision-tree.html

NUTRITIONAL INFORMATION

www.eatright.org
www.choosemyplate.gov

PHARMACOLOGY HELP

http://www.nova.edu/optometry/pharmacy
http://nursingpharmacology.info/
http://web.utah.edu/umed/courses/year2/pharm/study/

RESUME AND INTERVIEW TIPS

http://www.resume-now.com/lp/rnarsmnurs.aspx?cobrand=RSMN&tag=1209211
    85946583&hitlogid=118244876&ref=9095&utm_source=PPCg&utm
    _medium=SEMK&utm_term=how+to+write+a+nursing+resume&
    utm_campaign=e-Nursing

STRESS MANAGEMENT
http://helpguide.org/mental/stress_management_relief_coping.htm
http://holistic-online.com/Stress/stress_home.htm

STUDY AIDS
http://www.studygs.net
http://www.studystack.com/Nursing
http://www.howtostudy.org/resources_subject.php?id=31

■ ASSOCIATIONS

ALZHEIMER'S ASSOCIATION
http://www.alz.org

AMERICAN ASSOCIATION OF DIABETES EDUCATORS
www.diabeteseducator.org

AMERICAN CANCER SOCIETY
www.cancer.org

AMERICAN DIABETES ASSOCIATION
www.diabetes.org

AMERICAN FOUNDATION FOR THE BLIND
http://www.afb.org/default.aspx

AMERICAN HEART ASSOCIATION
http://www.heart.org/HEARTORG/

AMERICAN LUNG ASSOCIATION
http://www.lung.org/

AMERICAN NURSES ASSOCIATION
www.nursingworld.org

ARTHRITIS FOUNDATION
www.arthritis.org

BRAIN INJURY ASSOCIATION OF AMERICA
www.biausa.org

CYSTIC FIBROSIS FOUNDATION
www.cff.org

DEAFNESS RESEARCH FOUNDATION
www.drf.org

ENDOMETRIOSIS ASSOCIATION
www.endometriosisassn.org

EPILEPSY FOUNDATION
http://www.epilepsy.com/

HOSPICE AND PALLIATIVE NURSES ASSOCIATION
http://advancingexpertcare.org/

LEUKEMIA & LYMPHOMA SOCIETY
www.lls.org/

MULTIPLE SCLEROSIS ASSOCIATION OF AMERICA
www.msassociation.org

NATIONAL ASSOCIATION FOR CONTINENCE
www.nafc.org

NATIONAL ASSOCIATION FOR PRACTICAL NURSE EDUCATION AND SERVICE
http://napnes.org/drupal-7.4/

NATIONAL FEDERATION OF LICENSED PRACTICAL NURSES
www.nflpn.org

NATIONAL HEADACHE FOUNDATION
www.headaches.org

NATIONAL HEART, LUNG, AND BLOOD INSTITUTE
www.nhlbi.nih.gov

NATIONAL INSTITUTE OF ARTHRITIS AND MUSCULOSKELETAL AND SKIN DISEASES
www.niams.nih.gov

NATIONAL INSTITUTE ON AGING
www.nia.nih.gov

NATIONAL INSTITUTES OF HEALTH
www.nih.gov

NATIONAL KIDNEY FOUNDATION
www.kidney.org

NATIONAL MULTIPLE SCLEROSIS SOCIETY
www.nationalmssociety.org

NATIONAL PARKINSON FOUNDATION
www.parkinson.org

NATIONAL SLEEP FOUNDATION
www.sleepfoundation.org

THE NATIONAL SPINAL CORD INJURY ASSOCIATION
www.spinalcord.org

NATIONAL STROKE ASSOCIATION
www.stroke.org

NATIONAL STUDENT NURSES ASSOCIATION
www.nsna.org

THE NORTH AMERICAN MENOPAUSE SOCIETY
www.menopause.org

PARKINSON'S DISEASE FOUNDATION
www.pdf.org

SIMON FOUNDATION FOR CONTINENCE
www.simonfoundation.org

UNITED OSTOMY ASSOCIATIONS OF AMERICA, INC
www.ostomy.org

U.S. DEPARTMENT OF HEALTH AND HUMAN SERVICES OFFICE
ON WOMEN'S HEALTH
http://www.womenshealth.gov/

■ DRUGS AND NUTRITION RESOURCES

DRUGS, HERBS, AND SUPPLEMENTS
www.accessdata.fda.gov/Scripts/cder/DrugsatFDA
www.cancer.gov/cancertopics/druginfo/alphalist
www.drugs.com
www.drugwatch.com
http://nccam.nih.gov/health/herbsataglance.htm
www.nlm.nih.gov/medlineplus/druginformation.html

GLUTEN-FREE DIET
www.medicine.virginia.edu/clinical/departments/medicine/divisions/digestive
    -health/nutrition-support-team/nutrition-articles/Sept0601.pdf

LACTOSE-FREE DIET
http://www.livestrong.com/article/88755-gluten-dairy-list/

SPECIAL DIETS AND RECIPES
www.celiac.com
www.recipelink.com/specialdiets.html
www.recipesource.com/special-diets/diabetic
www.recipesource.com/special-diets/gluten-free
www.recipesource.com/special-diets/vegetarian
www.glutenfreediet.ca
www.glutenfreepassport.com
www.bestbreadrecipes.com/glutenfree.htm

VITAMINS AND MINERALS
www.cdc.gov/nutrition/everyone/basics/vitamins
www.nlm.nih.gov/medlineplus/vitamins.html

■ CONTINUING EDUCATION

http://ce.nurse.com/Webinar
www.ceufast.com
www.meniscus.com/
http://search.medscape.com/news-search?newSearch=1&queryText=CE+for+nurses
http://nursingworld.org/MainMenuCategories/ThePracticeofProfessional
    Nursing/NursingEducation/ContinuingEducationforNurses
http://www.ahrq.gov/professionals/education/continuing-ed/index.html
www.rnceus.com
www.rn.org
http://www.westernschools.com/healthcare-professions/nursing

■ DISEASE INFORMATION

ARTHRITIS
www.arthritis.org
www.healingwell.com/arthritis

ASTHMA AND ALLERGIES
www.aaaai.org
www.aafa.org
http://www.mayoclinic.org/diseases-conditions/allergies/basics/definition/con
    -20034030
www.medicinenet.com/allergy/article.htm

CANCER
www.canceradvocacy.org
www.cancer.gov
www.cancer.org
www.oncolink.org/index.cfm

DEPRESSION
www.metanoia.org/suicide/depressed.htm
www.webmd.com/depression/default.htm
http://www.suicidepreventionlifeline.org/

DIABETES
www.diabetes.niddk.nih.gov
www.joslin.harvard.edu

GASTROESOPHAGEAL REFLUX DISEASE (GERD)
www.medscape.com/resource/gerd

HEARING DIFFICULTIES
www.deaflibrary.org
www.listen-up.org

Online Resources

HEPATITIS C
www.hepatitis.va.gov/
www.hepatitis-central.com/
www.hepcnet.net/
www.hcvadvocate.org/library/library.asp
www.hepC-connection.org

HIGH CHOLESTEROL
www.cdc.gov/cholesterol
www.dietaryfiberfood.com/cholesterol-high-avoid.php

HIV/AIDS
www.aidsinfo.nih.gov
www.specialweb.com/aids
www.thebody.com/index/hotlines/national.html

HOSPICE AND PALLIATIVE CARE
www.hospiceresources.net
www.growthhouse.org
www.medscape.com/resource/hospice
www.stoppain.org/palliative_care/default.asp

HYPERTENSION
www.bplog.com/Resources.asp
http://www.nhlbi.nih.gov/health/health-topics/topics/hbp/

INFECTION AND DISEASE CONTROL
www.cdc.gov
www.nlm.nih.gov/medlineplus/infectioncontrol.html

LABORATORY TESTS
www.labtestsonline.org

LOW VISION INFORMATION AND RESOURCES
www.beyondsight.com
www.freedomvision.net
www.lighthouse.org
www.lowvision.com
www.lowvision.org
www.nyise.org/lowvision.htm

MIGRAINES
www.americanmigrainefoundation.org
www.headaches.org
www.healingwell.com/migraines
www.webmd.com/migraines-headaches/default.htm

PAIN
www.theacpa.org
https://www.painedu.org/resources.asp

PARKINSON'S DISEASE
www.michaeljfox.org/index.cfm
www.nlm.nih.gov/medlineplus/parkinsonsdisease.html
www.webmd.com/parkinsons-disease/default.htm

■ PATIENT EDUCATION

http://familydoctor.org/familydoctor/en/diseases-conditions/high-blood
    -pressure/diagnosis-tests/using-an-ambulatory-blood-pressure-monitor.html
www.ucsfhealth.org/adult/edu/index.html
http://vsearch.nlm.nih.gov/vivisimo/cgi-bin/query-meta?v%3Aproject=medline
    plus&query=Patient+education+&x=0&y=0

PATIENT FINANCIAL ASSISTANCE
http://www.sutterhealth.org/about/ab_uninsured.html
http://www.patientadvocate.org/resources.php?p=482

■ POST-TRAUMATIC STRESS DISORDER

http://www.giftfromwithin.org/
http://www.nimh.nih.gov/health/topics/post-traumatic-stress-disorder-ptsd/index
    .shtml
http://www.ptsdalliance.org/resources.html
http://www.ptsd.va.gov/

■ SLEEP PROBLEMS

www.sleepassociation.org
www.sleepnet.com/insomnia2000.html
www.webmd.com/sleep-disorders/insomnia-resources

■ SPINE HEALTH AND BACK PROBLEMS

www.backpainreliefonline.com
www.lower-back-pain-answers.com
www.spine-health.com
www.spineuniverse.com

■ WOUND CARE

www.medicaledu.com/Default.htm
www.wocn.org

■ COMMON SEARCH ENGINES

www.ask.com
www.bing.com
www.excite.com
www.google.com
https://www.google.com/chrome/browser/
www.yahoo.com

Online Resources

■ HELP LINES AND LINKS

http://www.crisiscallcenter.org/crisisservices.html
http://www.crisissupport.org/crisis_line
http://www.suicidepreventionlifeline.org/
http://www.dahmw.org/
http://www.helpguide.org/articles/abuse/help-for-abused-and-battered-women
    .htm
http://www.thehotline.org/blog/get-help-today/
http://www.acf.hhs.gov/programs/fysb/resource/help-fv
https://www.childhelp.org/hotline/

■ CUMULATIVE INDEX TO NURSING AND ALLIED HEALTH

www.ebscohost.com/academic/cinahl-plus-with-full-text/

■ ENGLISH-AS-SECOND LANGUAGE RESOURCES FOR NURSING STUDENTS

http://www.cabrillo.edu/academics/esl/resources.html
http://www.hospitalenglish.com/
http://nursing.gwu.edu/esl-writing-resources
http://www.usingenglish.com/links/English_for_Special_Purposes/Medical
    _English/

■ EVALUATION OF INTERNET RESOURCES

http://owl.english.purdue.edu/owl/resource/738/01
http://www.sc.edu/beaufort/library/pages/bones/lesson5.shtml

■ MEDICAL AND NURSING JOURNALS

www.nejm.org
www.jama.ama-assn.org
http://journals.lww.com/ajnonline/pages/default.aspx
www.medscape.com/welcome/journals
http://journals.lww.com/nursing/Pages/default.aspx
http://www.madeincrediblyeasy.com/products/nursing-made-incredibly-easy

■ NATIONAL CENTER FOR HEALTH STATISTICS

www.cdc.gov/nchs

■ TABLET AND SMARTPHONE APPLICATIONS AND SOFTWARE

http://itunes.apple.com/us/genre/mobile-software-applications/id6020?mt=8
http://us.blackberry.com/apps-software/appworld
www.unboundmedicine.com/products

■ RESEARCH AND JOURNAL WEBSITES

http://www.search.com/search?q=nursing+journals
http://www.medpagetoday.com/
http://www.medscape.com/nurses
www.nursingconsult.com/php/224890100-2/home.html

■ SENIOR HEALTH

http://nihseniorhealth.gov
http://www.nia.nih.gov/

■ UNITED STATES NATIONAL LIBRARY OF MEDICINE

www.nlm.nih.gov

BIBLIOGRAPHY

ANA: *Code of Ethics for Nurses with Interpretive Statements*, Washington, DC, 2001, American Nurses Publishing.

Black JM, Hawks JH, Keene AM: *Medical-surgical nursing: clinical management for positive outcomes*, ed 8, Philadelphia, 2009, Saunders.

Bope ET, Rakel RE, Kellerman RD, editors: *Conn's current therapy 2012*, Philadelphia, 2012, Elsevier.

Brothers K, Davis C, Kelton D, Shuss S: Managing your digital work life, *Nursing Made Incredibly Easy!* 12(3): 6–10, 2014.

Brous E: Professional licensure: investigation and disciplinary action, *AJN* 112(11):53–60, 2014.

Bryant M: Cracking the code: successful strategies for studying, *Nursing* 42(8):16–17, 2012.

Bucks County Community College: Websites on study skills, 2014. Retrieved from: www.bucks.edu/student/perkins/learn/websitesfor studyskills/.

Chancellor J: Effective study habits for nursing students, *Nursing2013* 43(4): 68–69, 2013.

Chrisman J, Jordan R, Davis C, Williams W: Exploring evidence-based practice research, *Nursing Made Incredibly Easy!* 12(4):8–12, 2012.

Cichminski L, Bellomo TL: Why me? Bullying and the answer to an age-old problem, *Nursing Made Incredibly Easy!* 10(3):58, 2010.

Collins SB: From "distress" to "de-stress" with stress management, *Nurse.com* 24(5):74–79, 2011.

Davis C: Keep your leadership skills sharp, *Nursing Made Incredibly Easy!* 12(2):4, 2012.

Davis C, Landon D, Brothers K: Safety alert: Protecting yourself and others from violence, *Nursing2015* 45(1): 55–59, 2015.

deWit SC: *Clinical quick reference for medical-surgical nursing: concepts & practice*, Philadelphia, 2009, Saunders.

deWit SC, Kumagai C: *Medical-surgical nursing: concepts & practice*, ed 2, St Louis, 2013, Saunders.

deWit SC, O'Neill P: *Fundamental concepts and skills for nursing*, ed 4, St Louis, 2014, Saunders.

Dombrosky TA: Responding to verbal abuse, *Nursing* 42(11):58–61, 2012.

Drugs.com: *Gluten-free diet: What should I avoid eating and drinking while on a gluten-free diet?* 2014. Retrieved from: http://www.drugs.com/cg/gluten-free -diet-aftercare-instructions.html.

Habel M: Building nurse-physician relationships, *Nurse.com* 25(6): 28–33, 2012.

Hanna AF, Suplee PD: Don't cross the line: respecting professional boundaries, *Nursing* 42(9):41–47, 2012.

Hart TL: *Speedy Spanish for medical personnel*, Santa Barbara, CA, 1980, Baja Books.

Hart TL: *Speedy Spanish for nursing personnel*, Santa Barbara, CA, 1988, Baja Books.

High-alert medications: no margin for error, *Nursing* 42(8):10, 2012.

Hill SS, Howlett HS: *Success in practical/ vocational nursing: from student to leader*, ed 7, St Louis, 2012, Saunders.

Hudson K: Safe medication administration—1 Nursing CE, DynamicNursingEducation.com, 2012. Retrieved from: http://dynamicnursingeduca tion.com/class.php?class_id38&pid= 15.

Ignatavicius DD, Workman ML: *Medical-surgical nursing: critical thinking for collaborative care*, ed 7, St Louis, 2013, Elsevier.

Institute for Safe Medication Practice: *ISMP list of error-prone abbreviations, symbols, and dose designations*, 2013. http://www.ismp.org/tools/error proneabbreviations.pdf.

Joyce EV, Villanueva ME: *Say it in Spanish: a guide for health care professionals*, ed 3, Philadelphia, 2004, Saunders.

Kee J, Hayes E, McCuistion L: *Pharmacology: a nursing process approach*, ed 7, St Louis, 2012, Elsevier.

Kirchner RB: Introducing nursing informatics, *Nursing2014* 44(9): 22–23, 2014.

Langford RW: *Mosby's PDQ for LPN*, ed 3, St Louis, 2013, Elsevier.

Laskowski-Jones L: The art of harmonious delegation, *Nursing Made Incredibly Easy!* 44(5):6.

Lee A: The role of informatics in nursing, *Nursing Made Incredibly Easy!* 12(4):55, 2014.

Lewis SL, et al: *Medical-surgical nursing: assessment & management of clinical problems*, ed 8, St Louis, 2011, Mosby.

Live Strong: *List of foods that contain lactose*. Retrieved from: http://www.livestrong.com/article/24875 -list-of-foods-that-contain-lactose/. Accessed July 22, 2012.

Mahan LK, Escott-Stump S, Raymond JL: *Krause's food, nutrition, & diet therapy*, ed 13, St Louis, 2012, Mosby.

Mayo Clinic Staff: Post-traumatic stress disorder (PTSD), 2014. Retrieved from: www.mayoclinic.org/ diseases-conditions/post-traumatic stress-disorder/basics/definition/ con-20022540.

McBride S, Delaney JM, Tietze M: Health information technology and nursing, *AJN* 112(8):36–42, 2012.

McCaffery M, Beebe A, Latham J: *Pain: clinical manual*, ed 2, St Louis, 1999, Mosby.

McCarron K: Routine labs for common meds, *Nursing Made Incredibly Easy!* 11(2):50–53, 2013.

Merritt S: Tips for computer-based multiple choice tests (CBT, CBE, and CAT), 2009. Retrieved from: http://masteringmultiplechoice .com/2009/09/tips-for-computer -based-tests- -cbt-cbe-and-cat/.

Miadowicz H: Biofeedback 101, *Nurse.com* 27(11):44–49, 2014.

National Institute of Mental Health: What are the symptoms of PTSD? 2014. Retrieved from: http:// www.nimh.nih.gov/health/topics/ post-traumatic-stress-disorder-ptsd/ index.shtml.

North American Nursing Diagnosis Association International: *Nursing diagnoses: definitions and classifications 2012-2014*, Philadelphia, 2012, The Association.

Northern Kentucky University: *Taking tests and quizzes* (online on Blackboard), 2014. Retrieved from: http:// pod.nku.edu/bb_student_test_asp.

Northwestern State University of Louisiana: *Test-taking tips for online exams*, 2014. Retrieved from: http:// ece.nsula.edu/test-taking-tips/.

Nugent PM, Vitale BA: *Test success: test-taking techniques for beginning nursing students*, ed 6, Philadelphia, 2012, FA Davis.

Nursing2013 Editors: Getting a grip on stress, *Nurse.com* 43(6):40, 2013.

Ortega L, Parsh B: Improving change-of-shift report, *Nursing2013* 43(2):68, 2013.

O'Toole MT: *Mosby's dictionary of medicine, nursing & health professions*, ed 9, St Louis, 2013, Mosby.

Pagana KD: Facebook: know the policy before posting, *Nurse.com* 24(6): 55–59, 2012.

Pagana KD: Mind your manners… multiculturally, *Nurse.com* 24(6): 49–51, 2012.

Pauk W, Owens RJQ: *How to study in college*, ed 10, New York, 2010, Cengage Learning.

Peckenpaugh NJ, Poleman CM: *Nutrition essentials and diet therapy*, ed 11, Philadelphia, 2010, Saunders.

Penn State Division of Undergraduate Studies: Study skills, 2014. Retrieved from: http://dus.psu.edu/academic success/studyskills.html.

Potter PA, Perry AG: *Fundamentals of nursing*, ed 8, St Louis, 2012, Mosby.

Potter PA, Perry AG, Ostendorf W: *Clinical nursing skills & techniques*, ed 8, St Louis, 2014, Mosby.

Rosati LJ: Strike gold when interviewing for your first nursing job, *Nursing2014* 44(5):49–52, 2014.

Sherman RO: Evidence-Based effective nursing leadership, *Nurse.com* 25(5): 68–73, 2012.

Smith LS: How to finance your dreams of further education. In *Lippincott's 2012 Nursing Career Directory*, Philadelphia, 2012, Wolters Kluwer/ Lippincott Williams & Wilkins, pp 28–33.

Strickler J: When it hurts to care: workplace violence in healthcare, *Nursing2013* 43(4):58–62, 2013.

Summers S: Sexually charged: how should a nurse respond when a patient makes inappropriate comments? *ADVANCE for Nurses* 2(10): 24, 2006.

Taylor S: Research reveals the benefits of meditation, *Nurse.com* 27(10): 36–41, 2014.

Texas Crime Watch: *Rape: ideas for self-protection*, pamphlet. n.d., Austin, Texas.

Tubesing DA: *Kicking your stress habits*, New York, 1981, Signet.

UCLA Department of Anesthesiology, David Geffen School of Medicine: *Universal pain assessment*. Retrieved: www.anes.ucla.edu/pain/in-dex.htm. Accessed February 9, 2009.

United States Department of Veterans Affairs: *Morse Fall Scale*, 2012. Retrieved from: http://www.patient safety.gov/cogAids/FallPrevention/ Index.html.

Williams SG: Back to school, *Advance for Nurses* 8(3):22–23, 2011.

Woods AD: Implementing evidence into practice, *Lippincott's 2013 Nursing Career & Education Directory*, 2013.

Zerwekh J, Garneau AZ: *Nursing today: transition and trends*, ed 7, Philadelphia, 2011, Saunders.

MAY 2016

SUNDAY	MONDAY	TUESDAY	WEDNESDAY	THURSDAY	FRIDAY	SATURDAY
1	2	3	4	5	6	7
8	9	10	11	12	13	14
15	16	17	18	19	20	21
22	23	24	25	26	27	28
29	30	31				

JUNE 2016

SUNDAY	MONDAY	TUESDAY	WEDNESDAY	THURSDAY	FRIDAY	SATURDAY
			1	2	3	4
5	6	7	8	9	10	11
12	13	14	15	16	17	18
19	20	21	22	23	24	25
26	27	28	29	30		

JULY 2016

SUNDAY	MONDAY	TUESDAY	WEDNESDAY	THURSDAY	FRIDAY	SATURDAY
					1	2
3	4	5	6	7	8	9
10	11	12	13	14	15	16
17	18	19	20	21	22	23
24	25	26	27	28	29	30
31						

AUGUST 2016

SUNDAY	MONDAY	TUESDAY	WEDNESDAY	THURSDAY	FRIDAY	SATURDAY
	1	2	3	4	5	6
7	8	9	10	11	12	13
14	15	16	17	18	19	20
21	22	23	24	25	26	27
28	29	30	31			

SEPTEMBER 2016

SUNDAY	MONDAY	TUESDAY	WEDNESDAY	THURSDAY	FRIDAY	SATURDAY
				1	2	3
4	5	6	7	8	9	10
11	12	13	14	15	16	17
18	19	20	21	22	23	24
25	26	27	28	29	30	

OCTOBER 2016

SUNDAY	MONDAY	TUESDAY	WEDNESDAY	THURSDAY	FRIDAY	SATURDAY
						1
2	3	4	5	6	7	8
9	10	11	12	13	14	15
16	17	18	19	20	21	22
23	24	25	26	27	28	29
30	31					

NOVEMBER 2016

SUNDAY	MONDAY	TUESDAY	WEDNESDAY	THURSDAY	FRIDAY	SATURDAY
		1	2	3	4	5
6	7	8	9	10	11	12
13	14	15	16	17	18	19
20	21	22	23	24	25	26
27	28	29	30			

DECEMBER 2016

SUNDAY	MONDAY	TUESDAY	WEDNESDAY	THURSDAY	FRIDAY	SATURDAY
				1	2	3
4	5	6	7	8	9	10
11	12	13	14	15	16	17
18	19	20	21	22	23	24
25	26	27	28	29	30	31

JANUARY 2017

SUNDAY	MONDAY	TUESDAY	WEDNESDAY	THURSDAY	FRIDAY	SATURDAY
1	2	3	4	5	6	7
8	9	10	11	12	13	14
15	16	17	18	19	20	21
22	23	24	25	26	27	28
29	30	31				

FEBRUARY 2017

SUNDAY	MONDAY	TUESDAY	WEDNESDAY	THURSDAY	FRIDAY	SATURDAY
			1	2	3	4
5	6	7	8	9	10	11
12	13	14	15	16	17	18
19	20	21	22	23	24	25
26	27	28				

MARCH 2017

SUNDAY	MONDAY	TUESDAY	WEDNESDAY	THURSDAY	FRIDAY	SATURDAY
			1	2	3	4
5	6	7	8	9	10	11
12	13	14	15	16	17	18
19	20	21	22	23	24	25
26	27	28	29	30	31	

APRIL 2017

SUNDAY	MONDAY	TUESDAY	WEDNESDAY	THURSDAY	FRIDAY	SATURDAY
						1
2	3	4	5	6	7	8
9	10	11	12	13	14	15
16	17	18	19	20	21	22
23	24	25	26	27	28	29
30						

MAY 2017

SUNDAY	MONDAY	TUESDAY	WEDNESDAY	THURSDAY	FRIDAY	SATURDAY
	1	2	3	4	5	6
7	8	9	10	11	12	13
14	15	16	17	18	19	20
21	22	23	24	25	26	27
28	29	30	31			

JUNE 2017

SUNDAY	MONDAY	TUESDAY	WEDNESDAY	THURSDAY	FRIDAY	SATURDAY
				1	2	3
4	5	6	7	8	9	10
11	12	13	14	15	16	17
18	19	20	21	22	23	24
25	26	27	28	29	30	

JULY 2017

SUNDAY	MONDAY	TUESDAY	WEDNESDAY	THURSDAY	FRIDAY	SATURDAY
						1
2	3	4	5	6	7	8
9	10	11	12	13	14	15
16	17	18	19	20	21	22
23	24	25	26	27	28	29
30	31					

AUGUST 2017

SUNDAY	MONDAY	TUESDAY	WEDNESDAY	THURSDAY	FRIDAY	SATURDAY
		1	2	3	4	5
6	7	8	9	10	11	12
13	14	15	16	17	18	19
20	21	22	23	24	25	26
27	28	29	30	31		

SEPTEMBER 2017

SUNDAY	MONDAY	TUESDAY	WEDNESDAY	THURSDAY	FRIDAY	SATURDAY
					1	2
3	4	5	6	7	8	9
10	11	12	13	14	15	16
17	18	19	20	21	22	23
24	25	26	27	28	29	30

OCTOBER 2017

SUNDAY	MONDAY	TUESDAY	WEDNESDAY	THURSDAY	FRIDAY	SATURDAY
1	2	3	4	5	6	7
8	9	10	11	12	13	14
15	16	17	18	19	20	21
22	23	24	25	26	27	28
29	30	31				

NOVEMBER 2017

SUNDAY	MONDAY	TUESDAY	WEDNESDAY	THURSDAY	FRIDAY	SATURDAY
			1	2	3	4
5	6	7	8	9	10	11
12	13	14	15	16	17	18
19	20	21	22	23	24	25
26	27	28	29	30		

DECEMBER 2017

SUNDAY	MONDAY	TUESDAY	WEDNESDAY	THURSDAY	FRIDAY	SATURDAY
					1	2
3	4	5	6	7	8	9
10	11	12	13	14	15	16
17	18	19	20	21	22	23
24	25	26	27	28	29	30
31						

MONDAY **APRIL 25**

TUESDAY **APRIL 26**

WEDNESDAY **APRIL 27**

THURSDAY **APRIL 28**

FRIDAY **APRIL 29**

SATURDAY **APRIL 30**

SUNDAY **MAY 1**

Weekly Planner

MAY 2-8   2016

MONDAY **MAY 2**

TUESDAY **MAY 3**

WEDNESDAY **MAY 4**

THURSDAY **MAY 5**

FRIDAY **MAY 6**

SATURDAY **MAY 7**

SUNDAY **MAY 8**

MAY 9-15 2016

MONDAY **MAY 9**

TUESDAY **MAY 10**

WEDNESDAY **MAY 11**

THURSDAY **MAY 12**

FRIDAY **MAY 13**

SATURDAY **MAY 14**

SUNDAY **MAY 15**

MAY 16-22 2016

MONDAY **MAY 16**

TUESDAY **MAY 17**

WEDNESDAY **MAY 18**

THURSDAY **MAY 19**

FRIDAY **MAY 20**

SATURDAY **MAY 21**

SUNDAY **MAY 22**

MONDAY **MAY 23**

TUESDAY **MAY 24**

WEDNESDAY **MAY 25**

THURSDAY **MAY 26**

FRIDAY **MAY 27**

SATURDAY **MAY 28**   SUNDAY **MAY 29**

MAY 30-JUNE 5 2016

MONDAY **MAY 30**

TUESDAY **MAY 31**

WEDNESDAY **JUNE 1**

THURSDAY **JUNE 2**

FRIDAY **JUNE 3**

SATURDAY **JUNE 4**

SUNDAY **JUNE 5**

JUNE 6-12

MONDAY **JUNE 6**

TUESDAY **JUNE 7**

WEDNESDAY **JUNE 8**

THURSDAY **JUNE 9**

FRIDAY **JUNE 10**

SATURDAY **JUNE 11**

SUNDAY **JUNE 12**

MONDAY **JUNE 13**

TUESDAY **JUNE 14**

WEDNESDAY **JUNE 15**

THURSDAY **JUNE 16**

FRIDAY **JUNE 17**

SATURDAY **JUNE 18**

SUNDAY **JUNE 19**

JUNE 20-26 2016

MONDAY **JUNE 20**

TUESDAY **JUNE 21**

WEDNESDAY **JUNE 22**

THURSDAY **JUNE 23**

FRIDAY **JUNE 24**

SATURDAY **JUNE 25**

SUNDAY **JUNE 26**

JUNE 27-JULY 3 2016

MONDAY **JUNE 27**

TUESDAY **JUNE 28**

WEDNESDAY **JUNE 29**

THURSDAY **JUNE 30**

FRIDAY **JULY 1**

SATURDAY **JULY 2**

SUNDAY **JULY 3**

JULY 4-10

MONDAY **JULY 4**

TUESDAY **JULY 5**

WEDNESDAY **JULY 6**

THURSDAY **JULY 7**

FRIDAY **JULY 8**

SATURDAY **JULY 9**

SUNDAY **JULY 10**

JULY 11-17

MONDAY **JULY 11**

TUESDAY **JULY 12**

WEDNESDAY **JULY 13**

THURSDAY **JULY 14**

FRIDAY **JULY 15**

SATURDAY **JULY 16**

SUNDAY **JULY 17**

MONDAY **JULY 18**

TUESDAY **JULY 19**

WEDNESDAY **JULY 20**

THURSDAY **JULY 21**

FRIDAY **JULY 22**

SATURDAY **JULY 23**

SUNDAY **JULY 24**

Weekly Planner

JULY 25-31

MONDAY **JULY 25**

TUESDAY **JULY 26**

WEDNESDAY **JULY 27**

THURSDAY **JULY 28**

FRIDAY **JULY 29**

SATURDAY **JULY 30**

SUNDAY **JULY 31**

MONDAY **AUGUST 1**

TUESDAY **AUGUST 2**

WEDNESDAY **AUGUST 3**

THURSDAY **AUGUST 4**

FRIDAY **AUGUST 5**

SATURDAY **AUGUST 6**

SUNDAY **AUGUST 7**

Weekly Planner

AUGUST 8-14 2016

MONDAY AUGUST 8

TUESDAY AUGUST 9

WEDNESDAY AUGUST 10

THURSDAY AUGUST 11

FRIDAY AUGUST 12

SATURDAY AUGUST 13

SUNDAY AUGUST 14

AUGUST 15-21 2016

MONDAY **AUGUST 15**

TUESDAY **AUGUST 16**

WEDNESDAY **AUGUST 17**

THURSDAY **AUGUST 18**

FRIDAY **AUGUST 19**

SATURDAY **AUGUST 20**

SUNDAY **AUGUST 21**

AUGUST 22-28 2016

MONDAY **AUGUST 22**

TUESDAY **AUGUST 23**

WEDNESDAY **AUGUST 24**

THURSDAY **AUGUST 25**

FRIDAY **AUGUST 26**

SATURDAY **AUGUST 27**

SUNDAY **AUGUST 28**

AUG 29-SEP 4 2016

MONDAY **AUGUST 29**

TUESDAY **AUGUST 30**

WEDNESDAY **AUGUST 31**

THURSDAY **SEPTEMBER 1**

FRIDAY **SEPTEMBER 2**

SATURDAY **SEPTEMBER 3**

SUNDAY **SEPTEMBER 4**

SEPTEMBER 5-11 2016

MONDAY SEPTEMBER 5

TUESDAY SEPTEMBER 6

WEDNESDAY SEPTEMBER 7

THURSDAY SEPTEMBER 8

FRIDAY SEPTEMBER 9

SATURDAY SEPTEMBER 10

SUNDAY SEPTEMBER 11

SEPTEMBER 12-18   2016

MONDAY **SEPTEMBER 12**

TUESDAY **SEPTEMBER 13**

WEDNESDAY **SEPTEMBER 14**

THURSDAY **SEPTEMBER 15**

FRIDAY **SEPTEMBER 16**

SATURDAY **SEPTEMBER 17**

SUNDAY **SEPTEMBER 18**

SEPTEMBER 19-25 2016

MONDAY **SEPTEMBER 19**

TUESDAY **SEPTEMBER 20**

WEDNESDAY **SEPTEMBER 21**

THURSDAY **SEPTEMBER 22**

FRIDAY **SEPTEMBER 23**

SATURDAY **SEPTEMBER 24**

SUNDAY **SEPTEMBER 25**

MONDAY **SEPTEMBER 26**

TUESDAY **SEPTEMBER 27**

WEDNESDAY **SEPTEMBER 28**

THURSDAY **SEPTEMBER 29**

FRIDAY **SEPTEMBER 30**

SATURDAY **OCTOBER 1**

SUNDAY **OCTOBER 2**

OCTOBER 3-9   2016

MONDAY **OCTOBER 3**

TUESDAY **OCTOBER 4**

WEDNESDAY **OCTOBER 5**

THURSDAY **OCTOBER 6**

FRIDAY **OCTOBER 7**

SATURDAY **OCTOBER 8**

SUNDAY **OCTOBER 9**

OCTOBER 10-16 2016

MONDAY **OCTOBER 10**

TUESDAY **OCTOBER 11**

WEDNESDAY **OCTOBER 12**

THURSDAY **OCTOBER 13**

FRIDAY **OCTOBER 14**

SATURDAY **OCTOBER 15**

SUNDAY **OCTOBER 16**

OCTOBER 17-23 2016

MONDAY **OCTOBER 17**

TUESDAY **OCTOBER 18**

WEDNESDAY **OCTOBER 19**

THURSDAY **OCTOBER 20**

FRIDAY **OCTOBER 21**

SATURDAY **OCTOBER 22**

SUNDAY **OCTOBER 23**

OCTOBER 24-30 2016

MONDAY OCTOBER 24

TUESDAY OCTOBER 25

WEDNESDAY OCTOBER 26

THURSDAY OCTOBER 27

FRIDAY OCTOBER 28

SATURDAY OCTOBER 29

SUNDAY OCTOBER 30

OCT 31-NOV 6 2016

MONDAY **OCTOBER 31**

TUESDAY **NOVEMBER 1**

WEDNESDAY **NOVEMBER 2**

THURSDAY **NOVEMBER 3**

FRIDAY **NOVEMBER 4**

SATURDAY **NOVEMBER 5**

SUNDAY **NOVEMBER 6**

NOVEMBER 7-13 2016

MONDAY **NOVEMBER 7**

TUESDAY **NOVEMBER 8**

WEDNESDAY **NOVEMBER 9**

THURSDAY **NOVEMBER 10**

FRIDAY **NOVEMBER 11**

SATURDAY **NOVEMBER 12**

SUNDAY **NOVEMBER 13**

NOVEMBER 14-20 2016

MONDAY **NOVEMBER 14**

TUESDAY **NOVEMBER 15**

WEDNESDAY **NOVEMBER 16**

THURSDAY **NOVEMBER 17**

FRIDAY **NOVEMBER 18**

SATURDAY **NOVEMBER 19**

SUNDAY **NOVEMBER 20**

NOVEMBER 21-27 2016

MONDAY **NOVEMBER 21**

TUESDAY **NOVEMBER 22**

WEDNESDAY **NOVEMBER 23**

THURSDAY **NOVEMBER 24**

FRIDAY **NOVEMBER 25**

SATURDAY **NOVEMBER 26**

SUNDAY **NOVEMBER 27**

Weekly Planner

NOV 28-DEC 4 2016

MONDAY **NOVEMBER 28**

TUESDAY **NOVEMBER 29**

WEDNESDAY **NOVEMBER 30**

THURSDAY **DECEMBER 1**

FRIDAY **DECEMBER 2**

SATURDAY **DECEMBER 3**

SUNDAY **DECEMBER 4**

DECEMBER 5-11 2016

MONDAY **DECEMBER 5**

TUESDAY **DECEMBER 6**

WEDNESDAY **DECEMBER 7**

THURSDAY **DECEMBER 8**

FRIDAY **DECEMBER 9**

SATURDAY **DECEMBER 10**

SUNDAY **DECEMBER 11**

Weekly Planner

DECEMBER 12-18　　　　2016

MONDAY DECEMBER 12

TUESDAY DECEMBER 13

WEDNESDAY DECEMBER 14

THURSDAY DECEMBER 15

FRIDAY DECEMBER 16

SATURDAY DECEMBER 17

SUNDAY DECEMBER 18

MONDAY **DECEMBER 19**

TUESDAY **DECEMBER 20**

WEDNESDAY **DECEMBER 21**

THURSDAY **DECEMBER 22**

FRIDAY **DECEMBER 23**

SATURDAY **DECEMBER 24**

SUNDAY **DECEMBER 25**

Weekly Planner

DEC 26-JAN 1   2016-2017

MONDAY DECEMBER 26

TUESDAY DECEMBER 27

WEDNESDAY DECEMBER 28

THURSDAY DECEMBER 29

FRIDAY DECEMBER 30

SATURDAY DECEMBER 31

SUNDAY JANUARY 1

MONDAY **JANUARY 2**

TUESDAY **JANUARY 3**

WEDNESDAY **JANUARY 4**

THURSDAY **JANUARY 5**

FRIDAY **JANUARY 6**

SATURDAY **JANUARY 7**

SUNDAY **JANUARY 8**

Weekly Planner

MONDAY **JANUARY 9**

TUESDAY **JANUARY 10**

WEDNESDAY **JANUARY 11**

THURSDAY **JANUARY 12**

FRIDAY **JANUARY 13**

SATURDAY **JANUARY 14**

SUNDAY **JANUARY 15**

JANUARY 16-22 2017

MONDAY JANUARY 16

TUESDAY JANUARY 17

WEDNESDAY JANUARY 18

THURSDAY JANUARY 19

FRIDAY JANUARY 20

SATURDAY JANUARY 21

SUNDAY JANUARY 22

JANUARY 23-29 2017

MONDAY **JANUARY 23**

TUESDAY **JANUARY 24**

WEDNESDAY **JANUARY 25**

THURSDAY **JANUARY 26**

FRIDAY **JANUARY 27**

SATURDAY **JANUARY 28**

SUNDAY **JANUARY 29**

MONDAY **JANUARY 30**

TUESDAY **JANUARY 31**

WEDNESDAY **FEBRUARY 1**

THURSDAY **FEBRUARY 2**

FRIDAY **FEBRUARY 3**

SATURDAY **FEBRUARY 4**

SUNDAY **FEBRUARY 5**

FEBRUARY 6-12 2017

MONDAY **FEBRUARY 6**

TUESDAY **FEBRUARY 7**

WEDNESDAY **FEBRUARY 8**

THURSDAY **FEBRUARY 9**

FRIDAY **FEBRUARY 10**

SATURDAY **FEBRUARY 11**

SUNDAY **FEBRUARY 12**

MONDAY **FEBRUARY 13**

TUESDAY **FEBRUARY 14**

WEDNESDAY **FEBRUARY 15**

THURSDAY **FEBRUARY 16**

FRIDAY **FEBRUARY 17**

SATURDAY **FEBRUARY 18**

SUNDAY **FEBRUARY 19**

Weekly Planner

FEBRUARY 20-26 2017

MONDAY **FEBRUARY 20**

TUESDAY **FEBRUARY 21**

WEDNESDAY **FEBRUARY 22**

THURSDAY **FEBRUARY 23**

FRIDAY **FEBRUARY 24**

SATURDAY **FEBRUARY 25**

SUNDAY **FEBRUARY 26**

MONDAY **FEBRUARY 27**

TUESDAY **FEBRUARY 28**

WEDNESDAY **MARCH 1**

THURSDAY **MARCH 2**

FRIDAY **MARCH 3**

SATURDAY **MARCH 4**

SUNDAY **MARCH 5**

MONDAY **MARCH 6**

TUESDAY **MARCH 7**

WEDNESDAY **MARCH 8**

THURSDAY **MARCH 9**

FRIDAY **MARCH 10**

SATURDAY **MARCH 11**

SUNDAY **MARCH 12**

MONDAY **MARCH 13**

TUESDAY **MARCH 14**

WEDNESDAY **MARCH 15**

THURSDAY **MARCH 16**

FRIDAY **MARCH 17**

SATURDAY **MARCH 18**

SUNDAY **MARCH 19**

Weekly Planner

MARCH 20-26　　　2017

MONDAY **MARCH 20**

TUESDAY **MARCH 21**

WEDNESDAY **MARCH 22**

THURSDAY **MARCH 23**

FRIDAY **MARCH 24**

SATURDAY **MARCH 25**

SUNDAY **MARCH 26**

MONDAY **MARCH 27**

TUESDAY **MARCH 28**

WEDNESDAY **MARCH 29**

THURSDAY **MARCH 30**

FRIDAY **MARCH 31**

SATURDAY **APRIL 1**

SUNDAY **APRIL 2**

Weekly Planner

APRIL 3-9

MONDAY **APRIL 3**

TUESDAY **APRIL 4**

WEDNESDAY **APRIL 5**

THURSDAY **APRIL 6**

FRIDAY **APRIL 7**

SATURDAY **APRIL 8**

SUNDAY **APRIL 9**

APRIL 10-16   2017

MONDAY **APRIL 10**

TUESDAY **APRIL 11**

WEDNESDAY **APRIL 12**

THURSDAY **APRIL 13**

FRIDAY **APRIL 14**

SATURDAY **APRIL 15**

SUNDAY **APRIL 16**

APRIL 17-23

MONDAY **APRIL 17**

TUESDAY **APRIL 18**

WEDNESDAY **APRIL 19**

THURSDAY **APRIL 20**

FRIDAY **APRIL 21**

SATURDAY **APRIL 22**

SUNDAY **APRIL 23**

APRIL 24-30 2017

MONDAY **APRIL 24**

TUESDAY **APRIL 25**

WEDNESDAY **APRIL 26**

THURSDAY **APRIL 27**

FRIDAY **APRIL 28**

SATURDAY **APRIL 29**

SUNDAY **APRIL 30**

MONDAY **MAY 1**

TUESDAY **MAY 2**

WEDNESDAY **MAY 3**

THURSDAY **MAY 4**

FRIDAY **MAY 5**

SATURDAY **MAY 6**

SUNDAY **MAY 7**

MAY 8-14

MONDAY **MAY 8**

TUESDAY **MAY 9**

WEDNESDAY **MAY 10**

THURSDAY **MAY 11**

FRIDAY **MAY 12**

SATURDAY **MAY 13**

SUNDAY **MAY 14**

MONDAY **MAY 15**

TUESDAY **MAY 16**

WEDNESDAY **MAY 17**

THURSDAY **MAY 18**

FRIDAY **MAY 19**

SATURDAY **MAY 20**

SUNDAY **MAY 21**

MONDAY **MAY 22**

TUESDAY **MAY 23**

WEDNESDAY **MAY 24**

THURSDAY **MAY 25**

FRIDAY **MAY 26**

SATURDAY **MAY 27**

SUNDAY **MAY 28**

MAY 29-JUN 4 2017

MONDAY **MAY 29**

TUESDAY **MAY 30**

WEDNESDAY **MAY 31**

THURSDAY **JUNE 1**

FRIDAY **JUNE 2**

SATURDAY **JUNE 3**

SUNDAY **JUNE 4**

JUNE 5-11

MONDAY **JUNE 5**

TUESDAY **JUNE 6**

WEDNESDAY **JUNE 7**

THURSDAY **JUNE 8**

FRIDAY **JUNE 9**

SATURDAY **JUNE 10**

SUNDAY **JUNE 11**

MONDAY **JUNE 12**

TUESDAY **JUNE 13**

WEDNESDAY **JUNE 14**

THURSDAY **JUNE 15**

FRIDAY **JUNE 16**

SATURDAY **JUNE 17**

SUNDAY **JUNE 18**

JUNE 19-25　　　　　　　　2017

MONDAY JUNE 19

TUESDAY JUNE 20

WEDNESDAY JUNE 21

THURSDAY JUNE 22

FRIDAY JUNE 23

SATURDAY JUNE 24

SUNDAY JUNE 25

JUNE 26-JULY 2 2017

MONDAY **JUNE 26**

TUESDAY **JUNE 27**

WEDNESDAY **JUNE 28**

THURSDAY **JUNE 29**

FRIDAY **JUNE 30**

SATURDAY **JULY 1**

SUNDAY **JULY 2**

JULY 3-9

MONDAY **JULY 3**

TUESDAY **JULY 4**

WEDNESDAY **JULY 5**

THURSDAY **JULY 6**

FRIDAY **JULY 7**

SATURDAY **JULY 8**

SUNDAY **JULY 9**

JULY 10-16 2017

MONDAY **JULY 10**

TUESDAY **JULY 11**

WEDNESDAY **JULY 12**

THURSDAY **JULY 13**

FRIDAY **JULY 14**

SATURDAY **JULY 15**

SUNDAY **JULY 16**

JULY 17-23 2017

MONDAY **JULY 17**

TUESDAY **JULY 18**

WEDNESDAY **JULY 19**

THURSDAY **JULY 20**

FRIDAY **JULY 21**

SATURDAY **JULY 22**

SUNDAY **JULY 23**

MONDAY **JULY 24**

TUESDAY **JULY 25**

WEDNESDAY **JULY 26**

THURSDAY **JULY 27**

FRIDAY **JULY 28**

SATURDAY **JULY 29**

SUNDAY **JULY 30**

JUL 31-AUG 6 2017

MONDAY **JULY 31**

TUESDAY **AUGUST 1**

WEDNESDAY **AUGUST 2**

THURSDAY **AUGUST 3**

FRIDAY **AUGUST 4**

SATURDAY **AUGUST 5**

SUNDAY **AUGUST 6**

MONDAY **AUGUST 7**

TUESDAY **AUGUST 8**

WEDNESDAY **AUGUST 9**

THURSDAY **AUGUST 10**

FRIDAY **AUGUST 11**

SATURDAY **AUGUST 12**

SUNDAY **AUGUST 13**

AUGUST 14-20 2017

MONDAY **AUGUST 14**

TUESDAY **AUGUST 15**

WEDNESDAY **AUGUST 16**

THURSDAY **AUGUST 17**

FRIDAY **AUGUST 18**

SATURDAY **AUGUST 19**

SUNDAY **AUGUST 20**

AUGUST 21-27 2017

MONDAY **AUGUST 21**

TUESDAY **AUGUST 22**

WEDNESDAY **AUGUST 23**

THURSDAY **AUGUST 24**

FRIDAY **AUGUST 25**

SATURDAY **AUGUST 26**

SUNDAY **AUGUST 27**

AUG 28-SEP 3   2017

MONDAY **AUGUST 28**

TUESDAY **AUGUST 29**

WEDNESDAY **AUGUST 30**

THURSDAY **AUGUST 31**

FRIDAY **SEPTEMBER 1**

SATURDAY **SEPTEMBER 2**

SUNDAY **SEPTEMBER 3**

SEPTEMBER 4-10 — 2017

MONDAY **SEPTEMBER 4**

TUESDAY **SEPTEMBER 5**

WEDNESDAY **SEPTEMBER 6**

THURSDAY **SEPTEMBER 7**

FRIDAY **SEPTEMBER 8**

SATURDAY **SEPTEMBER 9**

SUNDAY **SEPTEMBER 10**

SEPTEMBER 11-17   2017

MONDAY **SEPTEMBER 11**

TUESDAY **SEPTEMBER 12**

WEDNESDAY **SEPTEMBER 13**

THURSDAY **SEPTEMBER 14**

FRIDAY **SEPTEMBER 15**

SATURDAY **SEPTEMBER 16**

SUNDAY **SEPTEMBER 17**

SEPTEMBER 18-24 2017

MONDAY **SEPTEMBER 18**

TUESDAY **SEPTEMBER 19**

WEDNESDAY **SEPTEMBER 20**

THURSDAY **SEPTEMBER 21**

FRIDAY **SEPTEMBER 22**

SATURDAY **SEPTEMBER 23**

SUNDAY **SEPTEMBER 24**

SEP 25-OCT 1   2017

MONDAY **SEPTEMBER 25**

TUESDAY **SEPTEMBER 26**

WEDNESDAY **SEPTEMBER 27**

THURSDAY **SEPTEMBER 28**

FRIDAY **SEPTEMBER 29**

SATURDAY **SEPTEMBER 30**

SUNDAY **OCTOBER 1**

OCTOBER 2-8

MONDAY **OCTOBER 2**

TUESDAY **OCTOBER 3**

WEDNESDAY **OCTOBER 4**

THURSDAY **OCTOBER 5**

FRIDAY **OCTOBER 6**

SATURDAY **OCTOBER 7**

SUNDAY **OCTOBER 8**

OCTOBER 9-15 2017

MONDAY **OCTOBER 9**

TUESDAY **OCTOBER 10**

WEDNESDAY **OCTOBER 11**

THURSDAY **OCTOBER 12**

FRIDAY **OCTOBER 13**

SATURDAY **OCTOBER 14**

SUNDAY **OCTOBER 15**

OCTOBER 16-22 2017

MONDAY **OCTOBER 16**

TUESDAY **OCTOBER 17**

WEDNESDAY **OCTOBER 18**

THURSDAY **OCTOBER 19**

FRIDAY **OCTOBER 20**

SATURDAY **OCTOBER 21**

SUNDAY **OCTOBER 22**

OCTOBER 23-29 2017

MONDAY **OCTOBER 23**

TUESDAY **OCTOBER 24**

WEDNESDAY **OCTOBER 25**

THURSDAY **OCTOBER 26**

FRIDAY **OCTOBER 27**

SATURDAY **OCTOBER 28**

SUNDAY **OCTOBER 29**

MONDAY **OCTOBER 30**

TUESDAY **OCTOBER 31**

WEDNESDAY **NOVEMBER 1**

THURSDAY **NOVEMBER 2**

FRIDAY **NOVEMBER 3**

SATURDAY **NOVEMBER 4**

SUNDAY **NOVEMBER 5**

NOVEMBER 6-12 2017

MONDAY **NOVEMBER 6**

TUESDAY **NOVEMBER 7**

WEDNESDAY **NOVEMBER 8**

THURSDAY **NOVEMBER 9**

FRIDAY **NOVEMBER 10**

SATURDAY **NOVEMBER 11**

SUNDAY **NOVEMBER 12**

NOVEMBER 13-19 2017

MONDAY **NOVEMBER 13**

TUESDAY **NOVEMBER 14**

WEDNESDAY **NOVEMBER 15**

THURSDAY **NOVEMBER 16**

FRIDAY **NOVEMBER 17**

SATURDAY **NOVEMBER 18**

SUNDAY **NOVEMBER 19**

NOVEMBER 20-26 2017

MONDAY **NOVEMBER 20**

TUESDAY **NOVEMBER 21**

WEDNESDAY **NOVEMBER 22**

THURSDAY **NOVEMBER 23**

FRIDAY **NOVEMBER 24**

SATURDAY **NOVEMBER 25**

SUNDAY **NOVEMBER 26**

NOV 27-DEC 3   2017

MONDAY **NOVEMBER 27**

TUESDAY **NOVEMBER 28**

WEDNESDAY **NOVEMBER 29**

THURSDAY **NOVEMBER 30**

FRIDAY **DECEMBER 1**

SATURDAY **DECEMBER 2**

SUNDAY **DECEMBER 3**

MONDAY **DECEMBER 4**

TUESDAY **DECEMBER 5**

WEDNESDAY **DECEMBER 6**

THURSDAY **DECEMBER 7**

FRIDAY **DECEMBER 8**

SATURDAY **DECEMBER 9**

SUNDAY **DECEMBER 10**

Weekly Planner

DECEMBER 11-17　　　2017

MONDAY **DECEMBER 11**

TUESDAY **DECEMBER 12**

WEDNESDAY **DECEMBER 13**

THURSDAY **DECEMBER 14**

FRIDAY **DECEMBER 15**

SATURDAY **DECEMBER 16**

SUNDAY **DECEMBER 17**

DECEMBER 18-24 2017

MONDAY **DECEMBER 18**

TUESDAY **DECEMBER 19**

WEDNESDAY **DECEMBER 20**

THURSDAY **DECEMBER 21**

FRIDAY **DECEMBER 22**

SATURDAY **DECEMBER 23**

SUNDAY **DECEMBER 24**

DECEMBER 25-31 2017

MONDAY **DECEMBER 25**

TUESDAY **DECEMBER 26**

WEDNESDAY **DECEMBER 27**

THURSDAY **DECEMBER 28**

FRIDAY **DECEMBER 29**

SATURDAY **DECEMBER 30**

SUNDAY **DECEMBER 31**

INDEX

Page numbers followed by "f" indicate figures, "t" indicate tables, and "b" indicate boxes.